Table of Contents

Introduction

Alcohol consumption is deeply woven into the fabric of social culture, celebration, and even relaxation. However, what is often overlooked is the profound impact alcohol has on the body beyond the immediate effects of a buzz or hangover. This substance, while socially accepted, can wreak havoc on our biological systems, especially the intricate and delicate connection between the gut and the brain. Understanding these impacts is the first step toward making informed decisions about your health.

This book, *Dry January, Sober October: The Science Behind Cutting Alcohol Anytime*, is not just a guide to abstaining from alcohol for a set period. It is a deep dive into the science of how alcohol affects your body, particularly the gut microbiome—the diverse ecosystem of bacteria, fungi, and other microorganisms that play a crucial role in your overall health. Alcohol has a unique ability to alter this ecosystem, tilting the balance toward bad bacteria that can fuel cravings for more alcohol and sugar, setting off a cycle that can be difficult to break.

Through 30 individual case studies, we'll uncover the often-overlooked, far-reaching consequences of alcohol consumption. Each example highlights the biological mechanisms at play and the life-altering changes that occur when these mechanisms are disrupted.

One of the key areas of focus in this book is the gut-brain connection. The gut is often referred to as the "second brain" because of its direct communication with the brain via the vagus nerve and through chemical signals. Alcohol disrupts this communication, often leading to increased cravings for more alcohol or sugar. This disruption isn't just a matter of willpower; it's a physiological response driven by an imbalance in the gut microbiome. We'll explore how this imbalance can lead to a cascade of health issues, from mood disorders to metabolic disruptions.

Another critical topic covered in this book is how alcohol affects the body's ability to burn fat. Studies have shown that alcohol consumption halts fat oxidation for 24 to 48 hours. This means that while your body is processing alcohol, it prioritizes burning the alcohol-derived calories over other energy sources like fat. Over time, this can contribute to weight gain, inflammation, and metabolic issues. Understanding this process is key to recognizing why even moderate alcohol consumption can hinder health and fitness goals.

But this book isn't just about highlighting the problems; it's about offering solutions. You'll learn actionable strategies to reset your gut microbiome and restore a healthy balance of bacteria. We'll explore evidence-based methods for reducing cravings, improving mental clarity, and enhancing overall well-being. By the end, you'll have a comprehensive understanding of how alcohol affects your body and the tools to make informed decisions about your relationship with it.

Whether you're curious about participating in Dry January, Sober October, or simply exploring the idea of cutting back, this book is your guide to navigating the journey. It's about more than just temporary sobriety; it's about understanding the science behind your cravings and empowering yourself with knowledge to create lasting, positive changes in your health and lifestyle.

Alcohol and Gut Dysbiosis

Case Study #1: A study published in *Nature Microbiology* demonstrated that chronic alcohol consumption disrupts gut microbiota diversity, leading to an overgrowth of harmful bacteria like *Escherichia coli* while suppressing beneficial strains like *Lactobacillus*. This imbalance, or dysbiosis, impairs gut function and contributes to systemic inflammation.

The relationship between chronic alcohol consumption and gut health is a topic of increasing interest in scientific research, and for good reason. The gut, often referred to as the "second brain," plays a crucial role in overall health. It is home to trillions of microorganisms that make up the gut microbiota. This diverse ecosystem of bacteria, fungi, and other microbes is essential for digestion, nutrient absorption, immune function, and even mental health. When the balance of these microorganisms is disrupted, a condition known as dysbiosis occurs, which can have far-reaching consequences for the body. A study published in *Nature Microbiology* sheds light on how chronic alcohol consumption disrupts gut microbiota diversity, leading to an overgrowth of harmful bacteria like *Escherichia coli* while suppressing beneficial strains such as *Lactobacillus*. This imbalance impairs gut function and contributes to systemic inflammation, creating a cascade of negative health effects.

Understanding the Gut Microbiota and Its Importance

The gut microbiota is a complex and dynamic community of microorganisms that live in the digestive tract. This ecosystem includes beneficial bacteria, such as *Lactobacillus* and *Bifidobacterium*, which support digestion, produce vitamins like B12 and K, and help regulate the immune system. Harmful bacteria, such as *Escherichia coli*, are also present, but in healthy individuals, they are kept in check by the beneficial microbes. A balanced gut microbiota is crucial for maintaining intestinal integrity, preventing infections, and supporting overall health.

The composition of the gut microbiota is influenced by various factors, including diet, genetics, medications, and lifestyle choices. Alcohol consumption is one of the most significant lifestyle factors that can negatively affect gut health. Chronic alcohol use has been shown to reduce the diversity of gut microbiota, a marker of a healthy gut. Diversity in the gut microbiota is important because it allows for a wide range of functions, including breaking down complex carbohydrates, neutralizing toxins, and protecting against pathogens. When diversity is reduced, the gut's ability to perform these functions diminishes, making it more vulnerable to harmful bacteria.

The Impact of Alcohol on Gut Microbiota Diversity

Alcohol consumption, especially in chronic (daily) and excessive (binge) amounts, has a direct and detrimental impact on gut microbiota diversity. The study in *Nature Microbiology* revealed that chronic alcohol use creates an environment in the gut that favors the growth of harmful bacteria like *Escherichia coli*. *E. coli* is an opportunistic pathogen that can cause infections and produce harmful substances like lipopolysaccharides (LPS). LPS are toxins that can breach the gut lining and enter the bloodstream, triggering an immune response that leads to systemic inflammation.

At the same time, alcohol suppresses beneficial bacteria like *Lactobacillus*. *Lactobacillus* is known for its role in maintaining gut health by producing lactic acid, which lowers the pH of the gut environment and inhibits the growth of harmful bacteria. These beneficial bacteria also contribute to the production of short-chain fatty acids (SCFAs), which are essential for gut lining integrity and immune modulation. The suppression of *Lactobacillus* reduces the production of SCFAs, weakening the gut barrier and allowing harmful substances to leak into the bloodstream, a phenomenon known as "leaky gut."

Dysbiosis and Systemic Inflammation

Dysbiosis caused by chronic alcohol consumption doesn't just affect the gut; it has systemic repercussions. The overgrowth of harmful bacteria and the suppression of beneficial strains lead to increased permeability of the intestinal lining. This allows toxins like LPS and other microbial byproducts to enter the bloodstream, where they activate the immune system. While the immune response is designed to protect the body, chronic activation due to ongoing alcohol consumption leads to systemic inflammation.

Systemic inflammation is a key contributor to a range of chronic diseases, including liver disease, cardiovascular disease, and neurological conditions. In the case of alcohol-induced dysbiosis, the liver often bears the brunt of the damage. When toxins from the gut enter the liver through the portal vein, they can cause inflammation and damage liver cells, leading to conditions such as alcoholic hepatitis and cirrhosis. Additionally, systemic inflammation can affect the brain, contributing to cognitive decline and mental health issues such as depression and anxiety.

Long-Term Consequences of Gut Dysbiosis

The long-term consequences of alcohol-induced gut dysbiosis are profound. Beyond the immediate effects on gut function and systemic inflammation, chronic dysbiosis can weaken the immune system, making the body more susceptible to infections. It can also disrupt the gut-brain axis, the bidirectional communication network between the gut and the brain. This disruption has been linked to mood disorders, cognitive impairments, and even neurodegenerative diseases.

Furthermore, a compromised gut microbiota can lead to malnutrition. Chronic alcohol consumption impairs the gut's ability to absorb nutrients effectively, leading to deficiencies in vitamins and minerals that are essential for overall health. This malnutrition further exacerbates the negative effects of alcohol on the body, creating a vicious cycle of declining health.

Strategies to Restore Gut Health

The good news is that the gut has a remarkable ability to heal and regenerate when given the right support. Reducing or eliminating alcohol consumption is the first and most important step in restoring gut health. Abstaining from alcohol allows the gut microbiota to rebalance and regain its diversity.

Dietary changes can also play a significant role in supporting gut health. A diet rich in fiber, prebiotics, and probiotics can promote the growth of beneficial bacteria. Foods like yogurt, kefir, sauerkraut, and kimchi are excellent sources of probiotics, while fruits, vegetables, and whole grains provide prebiotics that feed beneficial bacteria. Additionally, incorporating fermented foods into the diet can help replenish beneficial bacteria and enhance gut diversity.

Supplementation may also be beneficial. Probiotic supplements containing strains like *Lactobacillus* and *Bifidobacterium* can help restore balance in the gut microbiota. Prebiotic supplements, which provide the nutrients beneficial bacteria need to thrive, can also support gut health.

Reducing stress and getting adequate sleep are other important factors in gut health. Stress and sleep deprivation can negatively affect the gut microbiota, exacerbating the effects of alcohol-induced dysbiosis. Practices like mindfulness, meditation, and regular physical activity can help reduce stress and support overall gut health.

The Role of Healthcare Professionals

Healthcare professionals play a vital role in addressing alcohol-induced gut dysbiosis. They can provide guidance on reducing alcohol consumption and offer personalized recommendations for restoring gut health. In cases of severe dysbiosis, medical interventions such as fecal microbiota transplantation (FMT) may be considered. FMT involves transplanting healthy gut bacteria from a donor to restore balance in the recipient's gut microbiota. While still a relatively new procedure, FMT has shown promise in treating severe cases of dysbiosis.

Alcohol has a profound impact on gut health, disrupting the delicate balance of the gut microbiota and leading to dysbiosis. This imbalance fosters the overgrowth of harmful bacteria like *Escherichia coli* while suppressing beneficial strains such as *Lactobacillus*, resulting in impaired gut function and systemic inflammation. The consequences of this disruption extend far beyond the gut, affecting the liver, immune system, brain, and overall health.

Understanding the connection between alcohol consumption and gut health highlights the importance of maintaining a balanced and diverse gut microbiota. By reducing alcohol intake, adopting a gut-friendly diet, and implementing lifestyle changes to reduce stress, individuals can support their gut health and mitigate the negative effects of alcohol. Healthcare professionals can provide valuable support and guidance in this journey, empowering individuals to take control of their health and well-being. Ultimately, protecting and nurturing gut health is a critical step toward achieving overall wellness.

Microbiome-Driven Sugar Cravings

Case Study #2: Researchers from the University of California found that alcohol-induced microbiome changes increase the production of short-chain fatty acids that signal the brain to crave sugar and alcohol, reinforcing addictive behaviors.

Researchers from the University of California have uncovered a fascinating and complex connection between alcohol consumption, the gut microbiome, and addictive behaviors. Their study revealed that alcohol-induced changes in the microbiome—the community of trillions of microorganisms living in the human digestive system—can directly influence brain function and behavior. These changes increase the production of specific substances called short-chain fatty acids (SCFAs), which act as chemical messengers between the gut and the brain. The increased levels of these SCFAs appear to play a significant role in signaling the brain to crave more sugar and alcohol, creating a feedback loop that reinforces addictive behaviors.

The gut microbiome plays an essential role in overall health, influencing everything from digestion and immunity to mood and cognition. However, its delicate balance can be disrupted by various factors, including diet, stress, medications, and alcohol consumption. Alcohol, in particular, has a profound and often harmful impact on the gut microbiome. Frequent or excessive drinking can kill off beneficial bacteria while allowing harmful bacteria to thrive. This imbalance, known as dysbiosis, can set off a chain reaction of negative effects throughout the body and mind.

One of the key consequences of alcohol-induced dysbiosis is the increased production of SCFAs, such as acetate, propionate, and butyrate. Under normal circumstances, SCFAs are produced during the fermentation of dietary fibers by beneficial gut bacteria and serve as an energy source for cells lining the gut. They also play a role in regulating inflammation and maintaining the gut-brain axis—a bidirectional communication system between the digestive system and the central nervous system. However, when alcohol disrupts the microbiome, the production of SCFAs becomes dysregulated.

Increased levels of SCFAs, particularly acetate, have been shown to directly influence the brain's reward and motivation centers. When these compounds enter the bloodstream, they can cross the blood-brain barrier and interact with neurons, triggering the release of dopamine—a neurotransmitter associated with pleasure and reward. This dopamine release can intensify cravings for substances that provide a similar reward, such as sugar and alcohol. In essence, *the gut is sending chemical signals to the brain that encourage behaviors reinforcing alcohol consumption and sugar intake.*

This process helps explain why individuals who consume alcohol frequently often develop strong cravings for sugary foods or drinks. Alcohol itself is a source of empty calories, and its consumption can lead to blood sugar spikes and crashes. The resulting low blood sugar levels further increase sugar cravings, creating yet another feedback loop. However, the role of the microbiome adds a deeper layer of complexity. By altering the microbiome and increasing SCFA production, alcohol consumption not only contributes to immediate cravings but also conditions the brain to associate alcohol and sugar with feelings of reward and satisfaction over the long term.

Understanding the role of the microbiome in reinforcing addictive behaviors is an exciting area of research, with significant implications for health and wellness. Addiction has traditionally been viewed as a condition driven primarily by psychological and genetic factors, but these findings highlight the importance of considering physiological and microbial influences as well. It suggests that treatments targeting the gut microbiome could provide a new avenue for addressing addictive behaviors. For instance, dietary interventions that promote a healthier balance of gut bacteria—such as increasing fiber intake, consuming probiotic-rich foods, or avoiding processed sugars—could potentially reduce SCFA dysregulation and help break the cycle of addiction.

Moreover, the study underscores the interconnected nature of dietary habits and alcohol consumption. Poor dietary choices, such as a high intake of processed and sugary foods, can compound the harmful effects of alcohol on the microbiome. These foods also feed harmful bacteria, further exacerbating dysbiosis. On the other hand, a balanced diet rich in whole foods, fruits, vegetables, and fermented products can support the growth of beneficial bacteria, enhancing the gut's resilience to alcohol-induced damage.

Additionally, researchers are exploring the potential of prebiotics and probiotics in addressing alcohol-related microbiome changes. Prebiotics are compounds that feed beneficial bacteria, while probiotics are live bacteria that can be introduced to the gut through supplements or fermented foods. Both have shown promise in restoring microbiome balance and reducing inflammation. However, more research is needed to determine how effective these approaches are in mitigating the specific effects of alcohol-induced dysbiosis.

Another fascinating aspect of this research is the potential influence of alcohol-induced microbiome changes on mental health. The gut and brain are deeply interconnected, and disruptions in the microbiome have been linked to a range of mental health issues, including anxiety, depression, and even cognitive impairments. By reinforcing addictive behaviors through the gut-brain axis, alcohol may also contribute to a cycle of emotional distress, where individuals turn to alcohol and sugar for temporary relief, only to experience worsening mental health in the long run.

The implications of these findings extend beyond individual health, shedding light on societal patterns of alcohol and sugar consumption. Both substances are highly prevalent in modern diets and are often consumed together, such as in cocktails, sugary mixers, or desserts. The combination may have a synergistic effect, reinforcing cravings and making it harder for individuals to moderate their intake. This insight emphasizes the importance of public health initiatives aimed at reducing the consumption of both alcohol and sugar while promoting gut-friendly dietary habits.

In practical terms, breaking the cycle of alcohol and sugar cravings involves a multifaceted approach. Reducing alcohol intake is a critical first step, as this allows the microbiome to begin recovering from the disruptive effects of alcohol. Incorporating microbiome-supporting foods, such as yogurt, kefir, sauerkraut, and fiber-rich vegetables, can further aid in restoring balance. At the same time, strategies to manage cravings—such as mindful eating, regular physical activity, and stress management—can help individuals regain control over their behaviors.

Finally, this research highlights the need for more education about the hidden ways alcohol affects the body. While most people are aware of its impact on the liver or its role in dehydration, few realize how profoundly it can influence gut health and, by extension, brain function and behavior. By raising awareness of these connections, researchers and health professionals can empower individuals to make more informed decisions about their consumption habits.

These findings provide valuable insights into how the gut and brain interact to shape cravings and behaviors, emphasizing the importance of gut health in addressing addiction. By taking steps to protect and restore the microbiome, individuals can break free from harmful cycles of alcohol and sugar consumption, paving the way for improved physical, mental, and emotional well-being. As research in this area continues to grow, it holds great promise for developing innovative strategies to combat addiction and promote overall health.

Alcohol and Leaky Gut Syndrome

Case Study #3: A 2017 study in *Gastroenterology* revealed that alcohol weakens the intestinal lining, allowing toxins and bacteria to leak into the bloodstream. This condition, known as leaky gut syndrome, triggers systemic inflammation and affects brain function.

In 2017, a pivotal study published in the journal *Gastroenterology* uncovered the profound effects of alcohol on the body, particularly its impact on the intestinal lining. The research highlighted how alcohol consumption weakens the protective barrier of the intestines, leading to a condition commonly referred to as leaky gut syndrome. This condition has far-reaching consequences for the body, including systemic inflammation and impaired brain function.

To understand how alcohol contributes to leaky gut syndrome, it's essential to first examine the role of the intestinal lining. The gastrointestinal (GI) tract is lined with a single layer of tightly packed epithelial cells, which act as a selective barrier. This barrier's primary job is to allow nutrients from digested food to pass into the bloodstream while keeping harmful substances like toxins, bacteria, and undigested food particles out. Tiny protein structures known as tight junctions hold these cells together, ensuring the integrity of the intestinal lining. When these tight junctions are compromised, gaps can form between the cells, allowing harmful substances to "leak" into the bloodstream. This phenomenon is what defines leaky gut syndrome.

Alcohol directly damages the cells lining the intestines and disrupts the tight junctions that maintain the barrier's integrity. When alcohol is consumed, it irritates the intestinal walls, leading to inflammation and oxidative stress. Over time, this repeated irritation weakens the tight junctions, making it easier for harmful substances to pass through the intestinal barrier. Additionally, alcohol promotes an imbalance in the gut microbiome—the diverse community of microorganisms that reside in the digestive tract. This imbalance, known as dysbiosis, further exacerbates the damage to the intestinal lining. Harmful bacteria proliferate, and beneficial bacteria that normally help maintain gut health and strengthen the intestinal barrier become depleted.

The consequences of leaky gut syndrome extend far beyond the digestive system. When toxins and bacteria enter the bloodstream, they can trigger a widespread inflammatory response. The body's immune system perceives these substances as threats and activates inflammatory pathways to neutralize them. While inflammation is a natural and necessary part of the immune response, chronic inflammation—such as that caused by a persistently leaky gut—can have devastating effects on overall health. Systemic inflammation has been linked to a range of chronic conditions, including heart disease, diabetes, autoimmune disorders, and even certain cancers.

One of the most concerning effects of systemic inflammation is its impact on brain function. The brain and gut are intricately connected through a communication network known as the gut-brain axis. This bidirectional pathway involves the nervous system, immune system, and endocrine system, allowing the gut and brain to influence each other's functions. When the gut becomes leaky and systemic inflammation occurs, inflammatory molecules and toxins can cross the blood-brain barrier—a protective membrane that normally prevents harmful substances from entering the brain. Once these substances breach the blood-brain barrier, they can disrupt neuronal function, impair cognitive processes, and contribute to neurodegenerative diseases such as Alzheimer's and Parkinson's.

The effect of alcohol-induced leaky gut on mental health is another critical area of concern. Studies have shown that systemic inflammation can alter the production of neurotransmitters—chemical messengers that regulate mood, behavior, and mental well-being. For example, chronic inflammation can reduce the availability of serotonin, often referred to as the "feel-good" neurotransmitter, leading to symptoms of depression and anxiety. Additionally, inflammation can increase levels of stress hormones like cortisol, which can exacerbate mental health issues and impair the body's ability to cope with stress.

Beyond the immediate effects on the gut and brain, leaky gut syndrome caused by alcohol consumption can have long-term implications for overall health. Persistent systemic inflammation places a significant burden on the body's organs and tissues, accelerating the aging process and increasing vulnerability to age-related diseases. Moreover, the disruption of the gut microbiome can weaken the immune system, making the body more susceptible to infections and illnesses. Research has also suggested that gut dysbiosis and leaky gut syndrome may play a role in the development of metabolic disorders such as obesity and insulin resistance, further compounding the health risks associated with alcohol consumption.

It is worth noting that the severity of alcohol's effects on the gut varies depending on factors such as the amount and frequency of alcohol consumption, individual genetics, and overall lifestyle. Heavy, chronic drinking poses the greatest risk for developing leaky gut syndrome and its associated complications. However, even moderate alcohol consumption can contribute to gut permeability and systemic inflammation, especially when combined with other factors such as a poor diet, stress, and lack of sleep.

Fortunately, the gut lining has a remarkable ability to heal and regenerate when given the right conditions. Reducing or eliminating alcohol consumption is one of the most effective ways to prevent and reverse leaky gut syndrome. Additionally, adopting a gut-friendly diet rich in whole, unprocessed foods can help restore the balance of the gut microbiome and strengthen the intestinal barrier. Foods high in fiber, such as fruits, vegetables, legumes, and whole grains, provide nourishment for beneficial gut bacteria, promoting a healthy microbial balance. Fermented foods like yogurt, kefir, sauerkraut, and kimchi are also excellent for replenishing beneficial bacteria.

Supplementing with nutrients and compounds that support gut health can further aid in the recovery process. For example, L-glutamine, an amino acid, plays a crucial role in maintaining the integrity of the intestinal lining and promoting healing. Probiotics, which are live beneficial bacteria, can help restore microbial balance and reduce inflammation. Omega-3 fatty acids, found in fatty fish, flaxseeds, and walnuts, have potent anti-inflammatory properties that can counteract the effects of systemic inflammation.

Managing stress and prioritizing sleep are also essential for gut health, as chronic stress and poor sleep can exacerbate gut permeability and inflammation. Practices such as mindfulness, yoga, and meditation can help reduce stress levels and improve overall well-being. Ensuring adequate hydration and avoiding other gut irritants like processed foods, excessive caffeine, and nonsteroidal anti-inflammatory drugs (NSAIDs) can further support the healing process.

The findings from the 2017 *Gastroenterology* study underscore the importance of understanding the far-reaching effects of alcohol on the body. While alcohol is often consumed for social enjoyment or relaxation, its potential to disrupt the delicate balance of the gut and trigger systemic inflammation cannot be overlooked. By recognizing the connection between alcohol, leaky gut syndrome, and overall health, individuals can make more informed choices about their alcohol consumption and adopt lifestyle habits that promote long-term well-being.

In conclusion, alcohol-induced leaky gut syndrome serves as a stark reminder of the intricate connections between the gut, immune system, and brain. The weakening of the intestinal lining caused by alcohol sets off a chain reaction of inflammation and dysfunction that impacts nearly every aspect of health. However, by taking proactive steps to minimize alcohol intake, nourish the gut, and support the body's natural healing processes, it is possible to mitigate these effects and pave the way for a healthier, more resilient body and mind. The key lies in making conscious choices that prioritize gut health as a cornerstone of overall wellness.

Inflammation and the Brain

Case Study #4: Inflammation caused by gut dysbiosis impacts the brain through the vagus nerve, contributing to mood disorders like anxiety and depression. A *Journal of Clinical Investigation* study showed a direct correlation between alcohol consumption, gut inflammation, and changes in brain chemistry.

The human body operates as a highly interconnected system, where the health of one part can significantly influence others. One of the most compelling examples of this is the relationship between gut health and brain health. Increasingly, scientific research is uncovering how gut dysbiosis—a condition where the balance of gut bacteria is disrupted—can contribute to inflammation that impacts brain function. This connection is largely mediated through the vagus nerve, a critical communication highway between the gut and the brain. The implications of this relationship are profound, particularly when it comes to mental health challenges like anxiety and depression.

The Role of the Vagus Nerve in Gut-Brain Communication

The vagus nerve plays a central role in the gut-brain axis, a bidirectional communication system that links the enteric nervous system in the gut with the central nervous system in the brain. The vagus nerve carries signals in both directions, allowing the gut and brain to share information about the body's physiological state. When the gut is healthy and its microbiota—the community of bacteria and other microorganisms living in the digestive tract—are balanced, this communication system works harmoniously. However, when gut dysbiosis occurs, the signals transmitted via the vagus nerve can become disrupted, leading to negative consequences for the brain.

Inflammation in the gut caused by an imbalance of harmful and beneficial bacteria triggers the release of pro-inflammatory cytokines. These molecules can travel along the vagus nerve, reaching the brain and causing neuroinflammation. This inflammation in the brain has been linked to altered neurotransmitter production and activity, which may contribute to mood disorders like anxiety and depression. Furthermore, gut dysbiosis has been shown to impair the production of short-chain fatty acids (SCFAs), which are critical for maintaining the integrity of the gut lining and regulating inflammation. Without sufficient SCFAs, the gut barrier becomes permeable—commonly referred to as "leaky gut"—allowing toxins and inflammatory agents to enter the bloodstream and exacerbate the cycle of inflammation.

Alcohol Consumption, Gut Health, and Mental Health

One significant contributor to gut dysbiosis is alcohol consumption. Alcohol is known to disrupt the delicate balance of gut bacteria by promoting the growth of harmful bacteria while reducing the population of beneficial ones. This imbalance leads to gut inflammation, which can profoundly affect brain chemistry. A study published in the *Journal of Clinical Investigation* highlighted the direct correlation between alcohol consumption, gut inflammation, and changes in brain function. This research provides valuable insights into how lifestyle factors like drinking can influence both physical and mental health.

Alcohol's impact on the gut extends beyond just altering the microbiota. It also damages the gut lining, increasing intestinal permeability and allowing harmful substances to enter the bloodstream. These substances, including bacterial endotoxins like lipopolysaccharides (LPS), can reach the brain and contribute to neuroinflammation. LPS has been shown to activate immune cells in the brain, leading to the release of inflammatory cytokines that interfere with normal brain function. This cascade of events can disrupt the production of key neurotransmitters such as serotonin and dopamine, which are critical for regulating mood.

Moreover, alcohol's effects on the gut and brain are cyclical. By promoting gut dysbiosis and inflammation, alcohol consumption can lead to feelings of anxiety and depression, which may, in turn, drive individuals to consume more alcohol as a coping mechanism. This creates a vicious cycle where gut and brain health deteriorate further over time.

Inflammation's Role in Anxiety and Depression

The link between inflammation and mood disorders is a rapidly growing area of research. While mental health conditions like anxiety and depression have traditionally been viewed through the lens of neurotransmitter imbalances, there is increasing recognition that inflammation plays a critical role in their development and progression. Inflammatory markers such as C-reactive protein (CRP) and interleukin-6 (IL-6) are often elevated in individuals with mood disorders, suggesting that systemic inflammation contributes to these conditions.

Gut inflammation, specifically, is a key driver of this process. When the gut is inflamed, the production of serotonin—a neurotransmitter often called the "feel-good chemical"—is disrupted. While serotonin is primarily associated with the brain, approximately 90% of the body's serotonin is produced in the gut. Gut dysbiosis and inflammation can reduce the availability of serotonin precursors, leading to lower serotonin levels in the brain and contributing to symptoms of anxiety and depression.

Additionally, inflammation affects the brain's reward pathways, which are responsible for feelings of motivation and pleasure. Chronic inflammation can impair the function of these pathways, leading to anhedonia, or the inability to experience pleasure—a common symptom of depression. This underscores the importance of addressing gut health not just for physical well-being, but also for emotional and mental health.

The Science Behind the Gut-Brain-Alcohol Link

The study from the *Journal of Clinical Investigation* provides robust evidence of how alcohol-induced gut inflammation impacts brain chemistry. Researchers observed that individuals who consumed alcohol regularly showed significant changes in the composition of their gut microbiota. These changes were accompanied by increased levels of gut-derived inflammatory markers in the bloodstream, which correlated with alterations in brain structure and function.

The study also highlighted the role of the vagus nerve in transmitting inflammatory signals from the gut to the brain. By stimulating the vagus nerve, researchers were able to mitigate some of the negative effects of gut inflammation on brain chemistry. This finding suggests that therapies aimed at improving vagus nerve function—such as mindfulness practices, vagus nerve stimulation devices, or dietary interventions—may hold promise for treating mood disorders linked to gut dysbiosis and alcohol consumption.

Practical Steps for Improving Gut and Brain Health

Addressing the impact of gut dysbiosis and inflammation on mental health requires a comprehensive approach. Diet is one of the most powerful tools for restoring balance to the gut microbiota. Consuming a diet rich in fiber, fermented foods, and prebiotics can help nourish beneficial bacteria and reduce inflammation. Avoiding alcohol or significantly reducing its consumption is also critical for protecting gut and brain health.

In addition to dietary changes, incorporating stress-management techniques can support the gut-brain axis. Chronic stress is known to negatively affect the gut microbiota, so practices like meditation, yoga, or deep-breathing exercises can help promote a healthier gut environment. Regular physical activity has also been shown to improve both gut and brain health by enhancing microbial diversity and reducing systemic inflammation.

Probiotic and prebiotic supplements may provide additional support for individuals with severe gut dysbiosis. Probiotics introduce beneficial bacteria into the gut, while prebiotics provide the nutrients these bacteria need to thrive. However, it is essential to choose high-quality supplements and consult a healthcare provider before starting any new regimen.

Finally, therapies that target the vagus nerve hold promise for improving gut-brain communication. Simple practices like humming, gargling, or even splashing cold water on the face can stimulate the vagus nerve and enhance its function. For individuals with more severe symptoms, medical devices that deliver electrical stimulation to the vagus nerve may be worth exploring.

The connection between gut health and brain health is a powerful reminder of how interconnected the human body truly is. Gut dysbiosis and the inflammation it causes can profoundly impact the brain through mechanisms like the vagus nerve, contributing to mood disorders such as anxiety and depression. Alcohol consumption exacerbates this issue by disrupting the gut microbiota and increasing inflammation, creating a harmful cycle that affects both physical and mental health.

Understanding and addressing this gut-brain connection is essential for improving overall well-being. By making dietary changes, managing stress, and exploring therapies that support the vagus nerve, individuals can take meaningful steps toward restoring balance to their gut and brain. As research continues to uncover the intricacies of the gut-brain axis, it becomes increasingly clear that prioritizing gut health is not just a trend but a fundamental aspect of holistic health care.

Alcohol Delays Fat Metabolism

Case Study #5: Alcohol is a toxin that the liver prioritizes metabolizing over fat and carbohydrates. Studies indicate that fat burning is suppressed for 24-48 hours after alcohol consumption as the liver focuses on detoxifying alcohol.

Alcohol is often seen as a harmless indulgence in social gatherings or as a way to unwind after a long day. However, when consumed, alcohol becomes a priority for the body to metabolize, pushing other critical processes like fat burning and carbohydrate metabolism to the back burner. This singular focus on detoxifying alcohol can significantly impact the body's ability to maintain a healthy balance, especially for those aiming to manage their weight or improve overall health.

When alcohol enters the body, it is treated as a toxin that requires immediate attention. Unlike macronutrients such as fats, proteins, and carbohydrates, which provide energy and essential nutrients, alcohol offers no nutritional benefit. Instead, it is metabolized by the liver, where enzymes such as alcohol dehydrogenase (ADH) and aldehyde dehydrogenase (ALDH) break it down into acetaldehyde and then acetate—both of which are further processed to prevent harm.

The liver's priority is to detoxify alcohol because of its potentially damaging effects on cells and tissues. This means that other metabolic processes, like the breakdown of fats and carbohydrates, are temporarily halted. The presence of alcohol in the bloodstream signals the liver to work overtime, ensuring that the toxin is processed and excreted as quickly as possible. Unfortunately, this prioritization comes at a cost to the body's overall metabolic efficiency.

Suppression of Fat Burning After Alcohol Consumption

One of the most significant consequences of alcohol metabolism is the suppression of fat oxidation. Studies have shown that fat burning is suppressed for 24-48 hours after alcohol consumption. This occurs because *the liver shifts its focus entirely to processing alcohol, leaving little to no capacity for metabolizing stored fats.*

During this time, the body enters a state where energy derived from dietary fats or fat stores is effectively put on hold. The liver produces acetate as a byproduct of alcohol metabolism, and this acetate becomes the primary fuel source during and after alcohol consumption. As a result, the body relies less on burning fats for energy and more on using acetate, which slows down weight loss efforts and may contribute to fat accumulation over time.

Moreover, alcohol consumption increases the likelihood of excess calories being stored as fat. Alcohol itself is calorie-dense, providing 7 calories per gram, and the metabolic shift it causes can exacerbate fat storage, especially in the abdominal area. This process highlights the connection between frequent alcohol intake and challenges in managing weight and body composition.

In addition to disrupting fat burning, alcohol consumption also affects carbohydrate metabolism and blood sugar regulation. Alcohol impairs the liver's ability to produce glucose through gluconeogenesis, which is critical for maintaining stable blood sugar levels. This suppression can lead to hypoglycemia, or low blood sugar, especially in individuals who drink on an empty stomach or engage in prolonged physical activity.

Furthermore, alcohol's impact on insulin sensitivity can have long-term consequences. Chronic alcohol consumption is linked to increased insulin resistance, a condition that makes it harder for cells to absorb glucose from the bloodstream. Over time, this can contribute to metabolic disorders like type 2 diabetes.

Beyond its immediate effects on fat and carbohydrate metabolism, alcohol consumption has broader implications for overall metabolic health. For instance, regular alcohol intake can disrupt hormonal balance, including hormones that regulate appetite and satiety. Alcohol stimulates the release of cortisol, a stress hormone, and lowers levels of leptin, the hormone responsible for signaling fullness. This combination can lead to overeating and a preference for calorie-dense, unhealthy foods.

Additionally, alcohol consumption can negatively affect the gut microbiome, a key player in overall health. The gut microbiome—a community of beneficial bacteria—is essential for digestion, immune function, and even mental health. Alcohol disrupts this delicate balance, promoting the growth of harmful bacteria while reducing beneficial strains. This imbalance can contribute to inflammation, poor nutrient absorption, and increased cravings for sugar and alcohol.

For those committed to improving their metabolic health, reducing or eliminating alcohol consumption offers numerous benefits. In addition to restoring the liver's ability to prioritize fat burning and carbohydrate metabolism, cutting back on alcohol can lead to better hormonal balance, improved insulin sensitivity, and a healthier gut microbiome. Over time, these changes can result in improved energy levels, enhanced weight management, and a lower risk of chronic diseases.

Moreover, reducing alcohol intake often brings mental health benefits, such as improved mood, better sleep quality, and reduced anxiety. These changes can create a positive feedback loop, where physical and mental well-being reinforce one another, making it easier to maintain healthier lifestyle habits.

Understanding the metabolic effects of alcohol underscores its impact as more than just empty calories. By prioritizing alcohol detoxification, the body temporarily sacrifices critical processes like fat burning and carbohydrate metabolism, leading to broader implications for weight management and overall health. For those seeking to optimize their metabolic function, reducing alcohol consumption is a powerful step toward achieving lasting health and wellness. Recognizing alcohol's role as a metabolic disruptor is key to making informed choices and fostering a healthier relationship with its consumption.

Increased Sugar Dependence

Case Study #6: A study in *Alcohol Research & Health* found that alcohol consumption disrupts dopamine pathways, heightening cravings for sugar as the body seeks quick energy replacements for alcohol's effects.

Dopamine is a neurotransmitter often referred to as the brain's "reward chemical." It plays a critical role in regulating pleasure, motivation, and reward-seeking behaviors. When we engage in enjoyable activities—such as eating, exercising, or socializing—dopamine levels increase, reinforcing those actions and encouraging us to repeat them. Alcohol consumption also triggers dopamine release, leading to the pleasurable effects many associate with drinking. However, this surge is temporary and disrupts the natural balance of dopamine pathways, leaving the brain in a deficit once the effects of alcohol wear off.

This study found that alcohol consumption interferes with dopamine pathways in a way that significantly impacts the body's energy regulation. Alcohol is metabolized in the liver, where it is converted into acetate, a quick source of energy. While this process provides an immediate energy boost, it disrupts the body's natural energy balance. When alcohol's effects subside, the body seeks to restore energy quickly, often by craving sugary foods. This happens because sugar, like alcohol, rapidly spikes dopamine levels, providing a temporary reward and energy boost. The brain essentially replaces one quick fix (alcohol) with another (sugar), creating a vicious cycle of cravings.

How Disrupted Dopamine Pathways Heighten Sugar Cravings

Alcohol's disruption of dopamine pathways does more than create a temporary energy deficit. It also alters how the brain perceives rewards. Over time, regular alcohol consumption can desensitize dopamine receptors, making them less responsive to natural sources of pleasure like food, social interactions, or exercise. This desensitization means that larger quantities of stimulants, like sugar, are required to achieve the same pleasurable effects. As a result, individuals who consume alcohol frequently may find themselves drawn to sugary foods and beverages to compensate for their reduced dopamine sensitivity. This effect is especially pronounced in individuals who consume alcohol regularly or in large amounts.

The Gut-Brain Axis and Alcohol-Induced Cravings

Another factor linking alcohol and sugar cravings is the gut-brain axis. This bidirectional communication system connects the gastrointestinal tract and the brain, playing a significant role in regulating appetite, mood, and overall health. Alcohol disrupts the gut microbiome, reducing populations of beneficial bacteria and allowing harmful bacteria to thrive. These harmful bacteria often feed on sugar and can influence the brain to crave more of it. Essentially, a disrupted gut microbiome caused by alcohol consumption can amplify sugar cravings through signals sent via the gut-brain axis. This cycle not only perpetuates cravings but also contributes to poor gut health, further exacerbating the problem.

Understanding the link between alcohol, dopamine, and sugar cravings is essential for breaking the cycle. Here are some effective strategies:

Focus on a Balanced Diet Eating a diet rich in whole foods, including vegetables, fruits, lean proteins, and healthy fats, can help stabilize blood sugar levels and reduce cravings. Incorporating complex carbohydrates, such as whole grains and legumes, provides sustained energy without the dopamine spikes caused by sugar.

Support Gut Health Probiotic-rich foods like yogurt, kimchi, and sauerkraut, as well as prebiotic foods like garlic and onions, can help restore a healthy gut microbiome. A balanced microbiome reduces the influence of harmful bacteria on sugar cravings.

Exercise Regularly Physical activity naturally boosts dopamine levels, helping to counteract the desensitization caused by alcohol. Even moderate exercise, such as walking or yoga, can improve mood and reduce cravings.

Hydrate and Rest Dehydration and lack of sleep can both increase cravings for quick energy sources like sugar. Drinking plenty of water and prioritizing quality sleep can reduce the intensity of cravings.

Mindful Practices Techniques such as meditation, deep breathing, or journaling can help manage stress, a common trigger for alcohol and sugar cravings. Stress management reduces the likelihood of turning to these substances for comfort.

Seek Professional Support If cravings feel unmanageable, seeking guidance from a nutritionist, therapist, or addiction specialist can provide tailored strategies for recovery and support.

Taking steps to reduce alcohol consumption and manage sugar cravings can have profound benefits for overall health. Breaking the cycle can improve dopamine function, restore gut health, and reduce the risk of conditions associated with excessive sugar intake, such as obesity, type 2 diabetes, and heart disease. It also supports better mental health, as stable dopamine levels and improved gut health are linked to reduced anxiety and depression.

By understanding the science behind alcohol's impact on dopamine pathways and sugar cravings, individuals can make informed decisions to improve their health and well-being. The journey may require effort and support, but the rewards—a healthier body, balanced energy levels, and improved mental clarity—are well worth it.

Reduced Bacterial Diversity

Case Study #7: Alcohol reduces the diversity of gut bacteria. A 2019 study in *Microbiome* highlighted that individuals who consume alcohol regularly have less diverse gut microbiota, a marker of poor health and immunity.

The relationship between alcohol consumption and gut health has gained significant attention in recent years, particularly as scientists uncover the intricate connections between the gut microbiome and overall health. One crucial finding is the impact of alcohol on the diversity of gut bacteria, an essential component of a healthy microbiome. A landmark 2019 study published in *Microbiome* revealed that individuals who consume alcohol regularly exhibit a marked decrease in gut microbial diversity, a key indicator of compromised health and weakened immunity. This discovery sheds light on the far-reaching consequences of alcohol use on the body, particularly through its influence on the gut.

What Is Gut Microbial Diversity and Why Is It Important?

The gut microbiome consists of trillions of bacteria, fungi, and other microorganisms that reside primarily in the digestive tract. These microbes play a vital role in digestion, nutrient absorption, and immune function. A diverse microbiome—one that includes a wide variety of beneficial bacterial species—is essential for optimal health. This diversity supports resilience against harmful pathogens, helps regulate inflammation, and even influences mental health through the gut-brain axis.

Reduced microbial diversity, on the other hand, has been linked to several health issues, including autoimmune diseases, obesity, diabetes, and depression. A well-balanced gut is like a thriving ecosystem, where each species contributes to the system's overall function. When alcohol disrupts this balance by reducing diversity, it creates a cascade of negative effects on physical and mental well-being.

This study highlighted a clear association between alcohol consumption and reduced gut microbial diversity. Researchers examined the gut microbiomes of individuals with varying levels of alcohol intake and found a significant difference between those who drank regularly and those who consumed little to no alcohol.

Regular alcohol consumption was linked to a decline in the abundance of beneficial bacterial species, including *Lactobacillus* and *Bifidobacterium*, which are known for their roles in digestion, immune support, and maintaining a healthy gut lining. At the same time, the study noted an increase in potentially harmful bacteria, such as *Enterobacteriaceae*, which are associated with inflammation and gut permeability (commonly referred to as "leaky gut").

These changes in the microbiome are concerning because they not only weaken the gut's defenses but also affect the body's ability to metabolize nutrients and maintain a balanced immune response. The researchers concluded that the negative effects on gut diversity were most pronounced in individuals who consumed alcohol consistently over time, suggesting that even moderate drinking could have long-term consequences for gut health.

The harmful effects of alcohol on gut health can be attributed to several mechanisms. First, alcohol is a known irritant to the gut lining. Chronic alcohol consumption damages the protective mucosal barrier in the intestines, allowing harmful substances and bacteria to enter the bloodstream. This process not only contributes to systemic inflammation but also creates an environment where beneficial bacteria struggle to thrive.

Second, alcohol has antimicrobial properties that can kill both good and bad bacteria. While this may seem like a double-edged sword, the reduction in beneficial bacteria often outweighs any temporary suppression of harmful microbes. Over time, the imbalance created by alcohol consumption disrupts the natural harmony of the gut microbiome.

Lastly, alcohol contributes to oxidative stress, a condition where the body produces an excess of free radicals that damage cells and tissues, including those in the gut. This oxidative damage further diminishes microbial diversity and impairs the gut's ability to heal itself, perpetuating a cycle of inflammation and dysfunction.

The Ripple Effect: Alcohol, Gut Health, and Immunity

One of the most concerning implications of reduced gut microbial diversity is its impact on the immune system. The gut houses nearly 70% of the body's immune cells, making it a critical component of immune defense. A diverse and balanced microbiome helps regulate immune activity, ensuring the body can fight off infections without overreacting to harmless stimuli.

When alcohol reduces microbial diversity, it weakens this regulation. Harmful bacteria may proliferate, triggering chronic inflammation that can overwhelm the immune system. This not only increases the risk of infections but also contributes to autoimmune disorders, where the body mistakenly attacks its own tissues.

Moreover, a compromised gut microbiome has been linked to reduced vaccine efficacy, slower recovery from illnesses, and heightened susceptibility to chronic diseases like heart disease and cancer. These findings emphasize the far-reaching consequences of alcohol-induced changes in gut health.

Can the Gut Recover from Alcohol's Effects?

The good news is that the gut microbiome is remarkably resilient, and positive changes in lifestyle can help restore its diversity. Reducing or eliminating alcohol consumption is a critical first step. Research shows that even short periods of sobriety, such as Dry January or Sober October, can lead to noticeable improvements in gut health and microbial diversity.

In addition to reducing alcohol intake, individuals can support their gut health through dietary changes. A diet rich in fiber, prebiotics, and probiotics can help replenish beneficial bacteria and encourage microbial diversity. Foods like yogurt, kefir, sauerkraut, and fermented vegetables are excellent sources of probiotics, while whole grains, fruits, and vegetables provide the prebiotics needed to nourish these microbes.

Other lifestyle factors, such as regular exercise, adequate sleep, and stress management, also play a crucial role in gut health. Studies have shown that physical activity can increase microbial diversity, while chronic stress and poor sleep can have the opposite effect.

Conclusion: Rethinking Alcohol's Impact on Health

The gut microbiome is a cornerstone of health, influencing everything from digestion and immunity to mental health and chronic disease risk. While occasional drinking may not cause significant harm for some individuals, regular alcohol consumption poses a clear risk to gut health by reducing microbial diversity and promoting inflammation. Understanding these risks empowers individuals to make informed choices about their alcohol intake and take proactive steps to support their gut microbiome.

By prioritizing gut health through a balanced diet, moderate or no alcohol consumption, and a healthy lifestyle, it is possible to protect this vital ecosystem and enjoy the wide-ranging benefits of a diverse and thriving microbiome.

Candida Overgrowth

Case Study #8: Alcohol feeds yeast such as *Candida albicans*, leading to overgrowth. This condition worsens gut health, increasing sugar cravings and perpetuating a vicious cycle.

Alcohol consumption has far-reaching effects on the human body, and one of the most significant yet often overlooked areas it impacts is gut health. The gut is home to trillions of microorganisms, collectively known as the gut microbiome, which play a critical role in digestion, immune function, and overall well-being. However, alcohol can disrupt this delicate ecosystem, paving the way for health issues, including Candida albicans overgrowth. This fungal imbalance not only worsens gut health but also fuels sugar cravings, trapping individuals in a harmful cycle.

The gut microbiome is a complex community of bacteria, fungi, and other microbes that coexist in a symbiotic relationship. When balanced, this system supports nutrient absorption, helps regulate metabolism, and strengthens the immune system. However, alcohol acts as a disruptor. When consumed, alcohol is absorbed through the stomach and small intestine, directly interacting with the gut lining and microbiota.

Studies have shown that even moderate alcohol consumption can lead to dysbiosis, a condition characterized by an imbalance in the gut microbiome. Alcohol decreases the population of beneficial bacteria such as Lactobacillus and Bifidobacterium while promoting the growth of harmful bacteria and fungi, including Candida albicans. This imbalance weakens the gut lining, making it more permeable—a condition commonly referred to as "leaky gut."

Candida albicans is a type of yeast that naturally resides in small amounts in the human body, including the gut. In a balanced microbiome, Candida is kept in check by beneficial bacteria. However, when the balance is disrupted, Candida can proliferate, leading to an overgrowth known as candidiasis.

Alcohol provides an ideal environment for Candida to thrive. First, alcohol contains sugars that feed yeast, enabling its rapid growth. Second, alcohol's inflammatory effects compromise the gut lining, reducing the immune system's ability to control Candida populations. As Candida overgrowth takes hold, it can cause symptoms ranging from bloating and fatigue to more serious issues like systemic inflammation and brain fog.

The Vicious Cycle of Alcohol and Sugar Cravings

One of the most insidious effects of Candida overgrowth is its ability to manipulate cravings. Candida thrives on sugar, and as it grows, it releases byproducts that signal the brain to crave more sugar and carbohydrates. Alcohol consumption exacerbates this cycle in multiple ways:

Alcohol Contains Sugar: Many alcoholic beverages are high in sugar, which feeds Candida directly. Even beverages that seem "dry" or low-sugar can still contribute to the problem because of alcohol's metabolism into acetaldehyde and other compounds that promote fungal growth.

Gut-Brain Axis Disruption: The gut and brain are intricately connected through the gut-brain axis. Candida overgrowth and alcohol-induced dysbiosis disrupt this communication, increasing cravings for sugar and alcohol.

Reduced Self-Control: Alcohol lowers inhibitions, making it harder to resist sugary foods and drinks, further feeding Candida and perpetuating the cycle.

Over time, this cycle becomes self-reinforcing, with each drink worsening gut health and increasing the body's dependency on sugar and alcohol for temporary relief.

Breaking the Cycle: Strategies for Recovery

Recovering from alcohol-induced gut issues and Candida overgrowth requires a multifaceted approach. Here are several strategies to help restore balance and break the cycle of cravings:

The first step in addressing Candida overgrowth is to eliminate its primary fuel sources: alcohol and sugar. Cutting out these substances starves the yeast and helps rebalance the gut microbiome. While this may be challenging at first, especially due to cravings, the long-term benefits far outweigh the temporary discomfort.

An anti-Candida diet focuses on whole, unprocessed foods that promote gut health. Key components include:

Non-Starchy Vegetables: Broccoli, spinach, and kale provide essential nutrients without feeding Candida.

Lean Proteins: Chicken, fish, and eggs support repair and recovery.

Healthy Fats: Avocados, nuts, and seeds help stabilize blood sugar levels.

Fermented Foods: Probiotic-rich foods like kimchi, sauerkraut, and kefir reintroduce beneficial bacteria to the gut.

Probiotics are beneficial bacteria that can help restore balance in the gut. Prebiotics, on the other hand, are non-digestible fibers that feed these good bacteria. Together, they create an environment hostile to Candida and conducive to healing.

As Candida dies off, it releases toxins that can cause temporary symptoms like headaches and fatigue, often referred to as "die-off" or Herxheimer reactions. Supporting the body's detoxification pathways can help mitigate these effects. Strategies include:

- Staying hydrated to flush out toxins.
- Supporting liver health with foods like leafy greens and turmeric.
- Engaging in gentle physical activity to promote lymphatic drainage

- Working with a healthcare provider, such as a naturopath or nutritionist, can provide personalized guidance and ensure that recovery efforts are safe and effective. Professionals can also recommend supplements like antifungal herbs or enzymes that specifically target Candida

Once the gut is healed, maintaining its health requires consistent effort. Key practices include:

- **Moderating Alcohol Consumption:** If reintroducing alcohol, do so sparingly and opt for low-sugar options like dry wine or spirits with no mixers.
- **Prioritizing Gut-Friendly Foods:** Continue incorporating fermented foods, fiber, and nutrient-dense meals into your diet.
- **Managing Stress:** Chronic stress can disrupt the gut microbiome. Practices like yoga, meditation, and deep breathing can help maintain balance.
- **Regular Exercise:** Physical activity supports gut health by promoting diverse microbiota and reducing inflammation.

The connection between alcohol, Candida overgrowth, and sugar cravings reveals a powerful truth: our dietary choices have profound implications for our health. While alcohol may seem like a harmless indulgence, its impact on the gut microbiome can set off a cascade of health challenges, from chronic inflammation to persistent cravings. Breaking the cycle requires commitment and lifestyle changes, but the rewards—improved energy, mental clarity, and overall well-being—are well worth the effort.

By understanding how alcohol affects gut health and taking proactive steps to restore balance, individuals can reclaim their health and break free from the grip of cravings. The journey to a healthier gut begins with informed choices, and every step toward better gut health is a step toward a healthier, more vibrant life.

Neuroinflammation

Case Study #9: The gut-brain axis is sensitive to microbiome changes. Alcohol-induced dysbiosis was shown to trigger neuroinflammation in a 2020 study, impacting cognitive functions like memory and decision-making.

The gut-brain axis refers to the intricate communication network that links your gut and brain. This bidirectional pathway involves multiple systems, including the central nervous system (CNS), the enteric nervous system (ENS), and the gut microbiome. It allows these systems to exchange information, regulating not only digestive processes but also cognitive and emotional functions. Emerging research underscores how the health of your gut can directly influence mental well-being, including mood, memory, and decision-making.

This connection is primarily facilitated by the gut microbiome, a diverse community of microorganisms living in your gastrointestinal tract. These microbes play essential roles in digestion, immune function, and the production of neurotransmitters like serotonin, often referred to as the "happy chemical." However, when the delicate balance of gut bacteria is disrupted, known as dysbiosis, the effects can ripple through the gut-brain axis, potentially leading to neuroinflammation and impaired cognitive functions.

Alcohol's Impact on Gut Microbiome Health

Alcohol consumption is a significant disruptor of gut health. When you drink alcohol, especially in excessive quantities, it can harm the lining of your gut and alter the composition of the microbiome. This process, known as alcohol-induced dysbiosis, involves a reduction in beneficial bacteria and an overgrowth of harmful ones. Such imbalances can weaken the gut barrier, allowing toxins and bacterial byproducts to enter the bloodstream, a condition referred to as leaky gut syndrome.

One of the most alarming consequences of alcohol-induced dysbiosis is its ability to promote systemic inflammation. When harmful bacteria flourish, they release endotoxins, which can trigger an immune response. Over time, this chronic inflammatory state may extend to the brain, a phenomenon known as neuroinflammation. Neuroinflammation has been linked to a host of mental health and cognitive issues, including anxiety, depression, memory loss, and difficulties with decision-making.

Neuroinflammation and Cognitive Decline

A 2020 study brought to light the profound connection between alcohol-induced dysbiosis and neuroinflammation. Researchers found that disruptions in the gut microbiome caused by alcohol led to increased levels of pro-inflammatory cytokines in the brain. These molecules are known to interfere with neural signaling and contribute to the degeneration of brain cells. Over time, this can impair cognitive functions such as memory, learning, and decision-making.

Memory, for instance, is highly dependent on the hippocampus, a region of the brain sensitive to inflammation. When inflammation takes hold, the hippocampus's ability to form and retrieve memories may be compromised. Similarly, decision-making relies on the prefrontal cortex, another area affected by neuroinflammation. Impairments in this region can lead to poor judgment and difficulty controlling impulsive behaviors, creating a vicious cycle where alcohol consumption becomes harder to manage.

Addressing alcohol-induced dysbiosis involves both reducing alcohol intake and actively supporting gut health. The gut microbiome is resilient and can recover with proper care. Here are some strategies to restore balance and protect the gut-brain axis:

Reducing Alcohol Consumption: Abstaining from or significantly reducing alcohol intake allows the gut lining to heal and gives beneficial bacteria a chance to repopulate.

Probiotic and Prebiotic Foods: Incorporating foods rich in probiotics, such as yogurt, kefir, and fermented vegetables, can help reintroduce healthy bacteria to the gut. Prebiotics, found in foods like garlic, onions, and bananas, provide the fiber that feeds these good bacteria.

Anti-Inflammatory Diet: Eating a diet rich in anti-inflammatory foods like leafy greens, berries, fatty fish, and nuts can reduce systemic inflammation and support gut health.

Regular Exercise: Physical activity has been shown to promote the growth of beneficial gut bacteria and enhance overall mental health.

Stress Management: Chronic stress can also disrupt the gut microbiome.

Practices such as mindfulness, yoga, and adequate sleep can help mitigate stress and improve gut health.

These steps not only aid in restoring the gut microbiome but also help reduce the risk of neuroinflammation, improving cognitive functions and emotional resilience over time.

Understanding the relationship between the gut-brain axis and alcohol consumption has profound implications for long-term health. Chronic alcohol use doesn't just impair immediate cognitive functions; it *may also increase the risk of serious neurological conditions like Alzheimer's disease and other forms of dementia.* This highlights the importance of maintaining a healthy gut microbiome as a preventive measure.

Moreover, the gut-brain axis's sensitivity to microbiome changes underscores the broader need for lifestyle choices that prioritize gut health. By fostering a balanced microbiome through diet, exercise, and stress management, you can not only protect your brain but also enhance your overall quality of life. This holistic approach is particularly critical for individuals recovering from alcohol dependency, as restoring gut health can play a pivotal role in breaking the cycle of addiction and promoting sustained recovery.

The gut-brain axis is a cornerstone of human health, acting as a vital link between our physical and mental well-being. Alcohol-induced dysbiosis disrupts this delicate balance, triggering neuroinflammation that can impair memory, decision-making, and emotional stability. However, the body's remarkable ability to heal offers hope. By making informed lifestyle choices, reducing alcohol consumption, and actively supporting gut health, it is possible to restore balance to the gut-brain axis and protect cognitive functions for the long term. This understanding empowers us to prioritize health and resilience in both mind and body.

Alcohol and Serotonin Production

Case Study #10: A healthy gut produces up to 90% of the body's serotonin. Alcohol disrupts this process by altering gut bacteria responsible for serotonin synthesis, contributing to mood disorders.

The human gut is more than just a digestive organ; it is a central hub for producing essential compounds that regulate overall health. Among its many functions, the gut plays a critical role in the synthesis of serotonin, a neurotransmitter often called the "feel-good chemical." Serotonin impacts mood, sleep, appetite, and even cognitive function. Remarkably, up to 90% of the body's serotonin is produced in the gut, underscoring the profound link between gut health and mental well-being. When the gut functions optimally, it fosters a delicate balance of bacteria that aids in serotonin production. However, alcohol consumption can disrupt this harmony, leading to far-reaching consequences for mental health.

The gut's ability to produce serotonin hinges on the symbiotic relationship between intestinal cells and gut bacteria. Specialized cells in the gut lining, known as enterochromaffin cells, synthesize serotonin using the amino acid tryptophan as a precursor. These cells do not work alone. They rely heavily on a thriving microbiome—the diverse community of bacteria, fungi, and other microorganisms residing in the gut—to facilitate this process. Certain beneficial bacteria, such as *Lactobacillus* and *Bifidobacterium* strains, are particularly important because they help regulate tryptophan metabolism and promote a gut environment conducive to serotonin production.

A healthy gut microbiome also communicates directly with the brain via the gut-brain axis, a bidirectional network of nerves, hormones, and immune signals. This communication ensures that serotonin and other mood-regulating chemicals are effectively distributed throughout the body, contributing to emotional stability and resilience.

Alcohol consumption, even in moderate amounts, can wreak havoc on gut health. It acts as a toxin that disrupts the balance of gut bacteria, favoring the growth of harmful microbes while suppressing beneficial ones. This phenomenon, known as dysbiosis, creates an inflammatory environment that damages the gut lining and impairs its ability to function properly. When the gut lining becomes compromised—a condition often referred to as "leaky gut"—toxins and undigested food particles can enter the bloodstream, triggering systemic inflammation.

Dysbiosis caused by alcohol not only hinders serotonin production but also affects the overall gut-brain axis. Without the right balance of bacteria, tryptophan is diverted away from serotonin synthesis and instead metabolized into other compounds that may exacerbate mood disorders. This disruption sets the stage for a range of psychological challenges, including anxiety, depression, and irritability.

Alcohol, Serotonin, and Mood Disorders

The connection between alcohol, gut health, and serotonin production explains why excessive drinking is often linked to mood disorders. People who consume alcohol regularly may notice short-term improvements in mood due to its initial sedative effects. However, these effects are deceptive and fleeting. *Over time, alcohol's interference with serotonin production can lead to mood instability and worsening mental health.*

Low serotonin levels have been directly associated with depression and anxiety. When the gut is unable to produce sufficient serotonin due to alcohol-induced dysbiosis, individuals may experience persistent feelings of sadness, hopelessness, or irritability. Furthermore, alcohol's impact on gut health may exacerbate stress levels by increasing cortisol, the body's primary stress hormone. Elevated cortisol further suppresses serotonin synthesis, creating a vicious cycle that can be challenging to break.

The good news is that the gut is remarkably resilient and can recover with proper care. Reducing or eliminating alcohol consumption is the first and most important step toward restoring a healthy gut microbiome. Once alcohol is removed, the body can begin the healing process, allowing beneficial bacteria to flourish and repairing the gut lining.

To support gut recovery and enhance serotonin production, consider the following strategies:

Incorporate Probiotics and Prebiotics: Probiotic-rich foods like yogurt, kefir, sauerkraut, and kimchi introduce beneficial bacteria into the gut. Prebiotic foods, such as bananas, garlic, and oats, provide the nourishment these bacteria need to thrive.

Eat a Balanced Diet: A diet rich in whole foods, fiber, lean proteins, and healthy fats supports gut health and provides the building blocks for serotonin synthesis. Including tryptophan-rich foods such as turkey, eggs, and nuts can further aid serotonin production.

Manage Stress: Chronic stress can negatively impact the gut-brain axis, so incorporating stress-reducing practices like meditation, yoga, or regular exercise can support both gut and mental health.

Stay Hydrated: Proper hydration supports digestion and helps maintain the gut's mucosal lining, which is essential for a healthy microbiome.

Understanding the interplay between alcohol, gut health, and serotonin production highlights the importance of adopting a holistic approach to health. Mental well-being is intricately tied to physical health, and the gut plays a pivotal role in bridging the two. By prioritizing gut health through mindful dietary and lifestyle choices, it is possible to not only restore serotonin levels but also improve mood, energy, and overall quality of life.

In conclusion, the gut's role in producing serotonin underscores its significance as a cornerstone of mental health. Alcohol disrupts this delicate process by altering the microbiome and impairing serotonin synthesis, contributing to mood disorders and other health challenges. However, with deliberate steps to reduce alcohol consumption and nurture the gut, it is possible to reclaim both physical and emotional well-being. By understanding and respecting the profound connection between the gut and the brain, individuals can unlock a powerful pathway to lasting health and happiness.

HPA Axis Dysregulation

Case Study #11: Chronic alcohol consumption dysregulates the hypothalamic-pituitary-adrenal (HPA) axis, leading to increased stress hormone levels. A disrupted HPA axis further impacts gut health and reproductive hormone balance.

Chronic alcohol consumption is known to wreak havoc on the hypothalamic-pituitary-adrenal (HPA) axis, one of the body's primary stress response systems. This complex network regulates the production and release of hormones, including cortisol, the body's main stress hormone. When functioning properly, the HPA axis helps maintain balance in the body by controlling processes such as metabolism, immune response, and mood regulation. However, prolonged alcohol use can dysregulate this system, leading to elevated levels of cortisol and other stress-related hormones. Over time, this dysregulation can have widespread effects on physical and mental health.

The mechanisms behind this disruption are multifaceted. Alcohol acts directly on the brain's hypothalamus, stimulating the release of corticotropin-releasing hormone (CRH). CRH signals the pituitary gland to produce adrenocorticotropic hormone (ACTH), which, in turn, prompts the adrenal glands to release cortisol. While occasional increases in cortisol are normal and even beneficial in response to acute stress, *chronic elevation due to alcohol misuse creates a persistent state of stress within the body.* This heightened stress state not only increases vulnerability to mental health conditions such as anxiety and depression but also impacts several other critical systems in the body.

Chronic Stress and Its Effects on Gut Health

One of the lesser-known consequences of HPA axis dysregulation is its impact on gut health. The gut and brain are intricately connected through the gut-brain axis, a bidirectional communication system that involves neural, hormonal, and immune pathways. Cortisol, when chronically elevated, disrupts this communication and can lead to a cascade of negative effects in the gastrointestinal system.

High cortisol levels weaken the integrity of the gut lining, leading to a condition commonly referred to as "leaky gut." In this state, the tight junctions between the cells of the intestinal lining become compromised, allowing toxins, pathogens, and partially digested food particles to enter the bloodstream. This triggers an immune response and promotes systemic inflammation, further exacerbating gut health issues.

Moreover, chronic stress from HPA axis dysregulation alters the composition of the gut microbiome, the diverse community of bacteria and other microorganisms that reside in the digestive tract. Alcohol exacerbates this imbalance by directly harming beneficial gut bacteria and promoting the growth of harmful species. This microbial imbalance, or dysbiosis, can lead to digestive issues such as bloating, diarrhea, and constipation. Additionally, dysbiosis has been linked to increased cravings for sugar and alcohol, creating a vicious cycle that perpetuates both alcohol consumption and gut health deterioration.

The Impact on Reproductive Hormones

The effects of a disrupted HPA axis extend beyond stress and gut health to include significant alterations in reproductive hormone balance. The HPA axis interacts closely with the hypothalamic-pituitary-gonadal (HPG) axis, which regulates the production of reproductive hormones such as estrogen, progesterone, and testosterone. When the HPA axis is dysregulated due to chronic alcohol consumption, this interaction becomes disrupted, leading to hormonal imbalances.

In women, elevated cortisol levels can suppress the release of gonadotropin-releasing hormone (GnRH) from the hypothalamus. GnRH is essential for stimulating the production of follicle-stimulating hormone (FSH) and luteinizing hormone (LH), which are critical for ovulation and the menstrual cycle. As a result, women who consume alcohol excessively may experience irregular menstrual cycles, reduced fertility, and other reproductive health issues. Prolonged HPA axis dysfunction can also contribute to conditions such as polycystic ovary syndrome (PCOS), which is characterized by hormonal imbalances and metabolic disturbances.

In men, chronic alcohol use and the associated HPA axis dysregulation can lead to decreased testosterone production. This occurs because elevated cortisol levels suppress the activity of the HPG axis, reducing the release of LH and, consequently, testosterone. Low testosterone levels can result in symptoms such as reduced libido, erectile dysfunction, and decreased muscle mass. Over time, these hormonal changes can significantly affect quality of life and overall well-being.

Mental Health Implications

The interplay between chronic alcohol consumption, HPA axis dysregulation, and mental health is profound. Elevated cortisol levels resulting from a disrupted HPA axis can increase susceptibility to mood disorders such as anxiety and depression. Cortisol directly affects brain regions involved in mood regulation, including the hippocampus and prefrontal cortex. Chronic exposure to high cortisol levels can impair the function of these brain regions, leading to cognitive deficits and emotional dysregulation.

Additionally, the gut-brain axis plays a critical role in mental health. Dysbiosis and leaky gut, both consequences of HPA axis dysfunction, can influence brain function through the release of pro-inflammatory cytokines and other signaling molecules. These inflammatory signals can cross the blood-brain barrier, contributing to neuroinflammation and exacerbating mental health symptoms. Thus, the combined effects of HPA axis dysregulation and alcohol's impact on the gut create a perfect storm for mental health challenges.

Addressing the effects of chronic alcohol consumption on the HPA axis and related systems requires a multifaceted approach. The first and most crucial step is reducing or eliminating alcohol intake. This allows the HPA axis to begin returning to its natural rhythm and helps lower cortisol levels. However, recovery from HPA axis dysregulation often takes time and requires additional supportive measures.

Stress Management Techniques: Incorporating practices such as mindfulness meditation, yoga, and deep breathing exercises can help reduce stress and support the HPA axis. These techniques promote relaxation and encourage the body to shift from a stress response to a state of rest and recovery.

Gut Health Support: A diet rich in fiber, fermented foods, and probiotics can help restore the gut microbiome. Avoiding processed foods, sugar, and other gut irritants is equally important. Supplements such as glutamine and zinc can support the repair of the gut lining and reduce inflammation.

Hormonal Balance: Working with a healthcare professional to address hormonal imbalances can be beneficial. This may involve dietary and lifestyle changes, as well as targeted supplementation to support reproductive health.

Mental Health Support: Counseling or therapy can provide valuable support for managing the emotional and psychological challenges associated with recovery. Cognitive-behavioral therapy (CBT) and other evidence-based approaches can help individuals develop healthier coping strategies and address underlying issues related to alcohol use.

Regular Exercise: Physical activity is a powerful tool for regulating cortisol levels, improving mood, and supporting overall health. Exercise also promotes a healthy gut microbiome and enhances the body's ability to handle stress.

The Long-Term Benefits of Restoring HPA Axis Function

By addressing the root causes of HPA axis dysregulation and implementing supportive lifestyle changes, individuals can experience significant improvements in their physical and mental health. Restoring balance to the HPA axis can lead to reduced stress, improved gut health, and normalized hormone levels. These changes, in turn, support better energy levels, enhanced mood, and overall resilience to life's challenges.

The journey to recovery may not be easy, but the rewards are well worth the effort. By understanding the interconnected effects of alcohol on the HPA axis, gut health, and hormonal balance, individuals can take proactive steps to reclaim their health and well-being.

Gut-Brain Signals and Addiction

Case Study #12: Research from the *American Journal of Psychiatry* found that alcohol alters gut-brain communication, enhancing addictive behaviors and reducing impulse control.

Research has unveiled critical insights into how alcohol consumption alters gut-brain communication. This interference not only enhances addictive behaviors but also impairs impulse control, creating a vicious cycle that fuels alcohol dependency. Understanding the gut-brain connection and the role alcohol plays in disrupting it is essential for addressing addiction and improving overall health.

The gut-brain axis is a complex communication network that links the gut and the brain via neural, hormonal, and immune pathways. This connection ensures that the brain and gut can share vital information about bodily functions, including digestion, mood regulation, and decision-making processes. The vagus nerve, a critical part of this axis, serves as a primary communication channel between the two systems. Additionally, the gut microbiome—a diverse community of microorganisms residing in the digestive tract—plays a pivotal role in maintaining gut-brain communication.

When this delicate balance is disrupted, as with alcohol consumption, the effects can extend beyond the digestive system to influence mental health, behavior, and decision-making abilities. Alcohol-induced alterations in this axis not only disrupt normal bodily functions but also set the stage for addictive tendencies and a loss of self-control.

One of the most significant ways alcohol affects the gut-brain axis is through its impact on the gut microbiome. *Alcohol is toxic to gut bacteria and can reduce the diversity and abundance of beneficial microbes.* These beneficial microbes are essential for producing short-chain fatty acids and neurotransmitters like serotonin, which regulate mood and behavior.

When alcohol disrupts the microbiome, harmful bacteria can proliferate, leading to gut inflammation and increased intestinal permeability, often referred to as "leaky gut." This condition allows toxins and harmful bacteria to enter the bloodstream, triggering an immune response that can affect the brain. Chronic inflammation caused by a disrupted gut microbiome has been linked to mental health disorders such as anxiety, depression, and, notably, addiction.

Enhanced Addictive Behaviors

The disruption of gut-brain communication by alcohol significantly enhances addictive behaviors. Research suggests that changes in the gut microbiome can alter dopamine signaling in the brain, the neurotransmitter responsible for feelings of pleasure and reward. With frequent alcohol consumption, the brain's reward system becomes hyperactivated, making it harder for individuals to resist cravings.

Moreover, alcohol alters the production of gamma-aminobutyric acid (GABA), a neurotransmitter that inhibits excessive neural activity and promotes calmness. Reduced levels of GABA, combined with an overstimulated reward system, create a perfect storm for addiction. These neurochemical changes, exacerbated by gut-brain axis disruption, make breaking free from alcohol dependence particularly challenging.

Impaired Impulse Control

Impulse control relies heavily on the prefrontal cortex, the area of the brain responsible for decision-making, self-regulation, and resisting temptations. Alcohol consumption has a direct impact on the prefrontal cortex, reducing its ability to function effectively. Simultaneously, disruptions in gut-brain communication amplify this effect by increasing inflammation and altering neurotransmitter production.

For example, the gut produces significant amounts of serotonin, often referred to as the "feel-good" hormone. When alcohol disrupts the gut microbiome, serotonin levels can drop, leading to mood swings, increased stress, and poor decision-making. This biochemical imbalance makes it more challenging for individuals to exercise restraint, further fueling the cycle of alcohol dependency.

Breaking the Cycle: Strategies for Restoring Gut-Brain Health

Given the profound impact of alcohol on the gut-brain axis, restoring this communication is a crucial step in overcoming addiction and improving overall health. Strategies for healing the gut-brain connection include:

Reducing Alcohol Consumption The first step in repairing the gut-brain axis is to minimize or eliminate alcohol intake. Abstinence allows the gut microbiome to begin healing and reduces the inflammatory processes triggered by alcohol.

Adopting a Gut-Friendly Diet A diet rich in fiber, fermented foods, and probiotics can help restore the diversity and balance of the gut microbiome. Foods such as yogurt, kefir, sauerkraut, and kimchi are excellent sources of beneficial bacteria. Additionally, prebiotic foods like garlic, onions, and bananas provide nourishment for these microbes.

Managing Stress Levels Chronic stress can further disrupt gut-brain communication. Practices such as mindfulness meditation, yoga, and regular physical activity can help reduce stress and support healthy gut function.

Using Probiotic and Prebiotic Supplements Probiotic and prebiotic supplements can help repopulate the gut with beneficial bacteria and promote a healthy environment for these microbes to thrive. Consulting with a healthcare provider can help determine the most effective options.

Seeking Professional Support For individuals struggling with alcohol dependency, professional support from addiction specialists, therapists, and support groups is invaluable. Addressing both the psychological and physiological aspects of addiction increases the likelihood of long-term recovery.

The Broader Implications for Mental and Physical Health

The relationship between alcohol and gut-brain communication extends beyond addiction. Chronic alcohol consumption has been linked to various health issues, including liver disease, cardiovascular problems, and neurological disorders. By disrupting the gut-brain axis, alcohol also contributes to mood disorders, cognitive decline, and impaired immune function.

Recognizing and addressing the impact of alcohol on the gut-brain connection can lead to improved mental clarity, emotional stability, and physical well-being. Research continues to explore this dynamic relationship, offering new insights into the role of gut health in addiction and overall health.

The findings from the *American Journal of Psychiatry* underscore the profound influence of alcohol on gut-brain communication. By disrupting the gut microbiome, altering neurotransmitter production, and impairing impulse control, alcohol sets the stage for enhanced addictive behaviors and long-term health consequences. Addressing these effects requires a comprehensive approach that includes reducing alcohol intake, supporting gut health, and seeking professional assistance when needed. Through these strategies, individuals can break free from the cycle of addiction and reclaim their health and well-being.

Impaired Nutrient Absorption

Case Study #13: Alcohol damages the gut lining, reducing absorption of critical nutrients like B vitamins and magnesium, which are essential for brain and metabolic health.

Alcohol consumption has long been associated with a variety of health concerns, and one of the most significant yet often overlooked areas of impact is the gut. The gut plays a crucial role in overall health, serving as the gateway for nutrient absorption and a key regulator of the immune system. When alcohol disrupts the gut, it can set off a cascade of negative effects that influence not only digestive health but also brain and metabolic function. Understanding how alcohol damages the gut and impairs nutrient absorption is vital for anyone seeking to improve their health and well-being.

The gut lining is composed of a delicate layer of cells that acts as a barrier, protecting the body from harmful substances while allowing essential nutrients to pass into the bloodstream. Alcohol can erode this lining by increasing the production of inflammatory molecules, such as cytokines, and disrupting the tight junctions between cells.

This condition, often referred to as "leaky gut," allows toxins and partially digested food particles to escape into the bloodstream, triggering systemic inflammation and a heightened immune response.

Over time, chronic alcohol consumption exacerbates this damage. It not only increases gut permeability but also alters the balance of gut microbiota. These changes contribute to an unhealthy gut environment, making it even more difficult for the gut lining to repair itself. As the barrier weakens, the body becomes less efficient at absorbing the nutrients needed for optimal health.

One of the most profound consequences of alcohol-induced gut damage is the reduced absorption of critical nutrients, including B vitamins and magnesium. These nutrients are essential for a variety of bodily functions, and deficiencies can have widespread effects on health:

B Vitamins: The Unsung Heroes of Brain Health

B vitamins, particularly B1 (thiamine), B6 (pyridoxine), B9 (folate), and B12 (cobalamin), are crucial for brain function, energy production, and red blood cell formation. Alcohol impairs the gut's ability to absorb these vitamins by damaging the cells responsible for transporting them into the bloodstream. This can lead to deficiencies that manifest as fatigue, cognitive decline, and mood disturbances.

For instance, a deficiency in thiamine can result in Wernicke-Korsakoff syndrome, a serious neurological condition often seen in chronic alcohol users. Folate and B12 deficiencies, on the other hand, are linked to anemia, depression, and impaired DNA synthesis, which can hinder cellular repair and growth.

Magnesium: The Metabolic Powerhouse

Magnesium is another nutrient frequently depleted by alcohol consumption. This mineral is vital for over 300 enzymatic reactions in the body, including those involved in energy production, muscle function, and nerve signaling. Alcohol disrupts magnesium absorption by increasing its excretion through the kidneys and reducing its uptake in the gut.

Low magnesium levels can lead to symptoms such as muscle cramps, irregular heart rhythms, and increased susceptibility to stress. Moreover, magnesium is critical for maintaining blood sugar stability and metabolic health. A deficiency can exacerbate conditions like insulin resistance, making it more difficult to manage weight and energy levels.

The Domino Effect: How Gut Damage Impacts Brain and Metabolic Health

The gut and brain are intricately connected through the gut-brain axis, a bidirectional communication network involving the nervous, immune, and endocrine systems. Damage to the gut lining and microbiome caused by alcohol consumption can disrupt this connection, leading to both cognitive and metabolic consequences.

Nutrient deficiencies caused by poor gut absorption can significantly affect brain function. B vitamins are essential for the production of neurotransmitters such as serotonin and dopamine, which regulate mood, focus, and energy levels. Without adequate levels of these vitamins, individuals may experience brain fog, anxiety, and depression.

Additionally, systemic inflammation stemming from a leaky gut can cross the blood-brain barrier, further contributing to cognitive and emotional challenges. This inflammatory response is a common factor in the development of neurological disorders, highlighting the critical need for gut health in maintaining mental clarity and emotional resilience.

The gut also plays a pivotal role in regulating metabolism, and alcohol-induced damage can interfere with this process. When the gut's ability to absorb magnesium and other nutrients is compromised, the body's metabolic machinery suffers. Magnesium deficiency, for example, can impair the production of adenosine triphosphate (ATP), the molecule that provides energy to cells. This can lead to fatigue and difficulty maintaining a healthy weight.

Furthermore, alcohol disrupts the balance of gut bacteria, reducing populations of beneficial microbes that help regulate blood sugar and fat storage.

This microbial imbalance, known as dysbiosis, can contribute to insulin resistance and increased fat accumulation, particularly around the abdomen.

To repair the gut lining, consider incorporating foods and supplements known for their gut-healing properties. Bone broth, rich in collagen and amino acids, can help strengthen the gut barrier. L-glutamine, an amino acid available as a supplement, is another excellent option for promoting gut health. Probiotics can also play a key role in restoring microbial balance and reducing inflammation.

The damage alcohol inflicts on the gut lining and nutrient absorption underscores the importance of moderating consumption and prioritizing gut health. By understanding the link between alcohol, nutrient deficiencies, and broader health outcomes, individuals can make informed choices to protect their well-being. With the right strategies, it is possible to heal the gut, restore nutrient levels, and enjoy improved brain and metabolic health.

Alcohol-Induced Insulin Resistance

Case Study #14: A *Diabetes Care* study found that alcohol consumption exacerbates insulin resistance, linking it to metabolic syndrome and weight gain.

In recent years, scientists have uncovered more about how alcohol consumption affects metabolic health. Understanding this connection is crucial for anyone aiming to maintain metabolic health or manage conditions such as diabetes, obesity, or cardiovascular disease.

Insulin resistance occurs when the body's cells fail to respond effectively to insulin, the hormone responsible for regulating blood sugar levels. Over time, this can lead to elevated blood sugar levels, prediabetes, and type 2 diabetes.

When you consume alcohol, your body prioritizes metabolizing it over other substances like glucose or fat. This happens because alcohol is treated as a toxin that must be eliminated. While the liver works to process alcohol, it temporarily halts its normal role in glucose and fat metabolism. This disruption increases insulin resistance by impairing the liver's ability to regulate glucose levels and influencing how fat is stored in the body.

Moreover, alcohol consumption can lead to chronic inflammation and oxidative stress, both of which are known to aggravate insulin resistance. These processes damage cells and tissues, making it harder for insulin to do its job. In individuals who already have a predisposition to insulin resistance, even moderate alcohol intake can have a cumulative effect, worsening the condition over time.

Metabolic syndrome is a cluster of conditions that includes high blood pressure, elevated blood sugar, abnormal cholesterol levels, and excess abdominal fat. This syndrome significantly increases the risk of type 2 diabetes, heart disease, and stroke. The *Diabetes Care* study highlights alcohol as a major contributor to the development and progression of metabolic syndrome.

One way alcohol contributes to metabolic syndrome is by altering the gut microbiome. Alcohol disrupts the balance of beneficial and harmful bacteria in the gut, leading to an increase in gut permeability. This condition, often referred to as "leaky gut," allows toxins and inflammatory compounds to enter the bloodstream.

These substances can interfere with insulin signaling and promote fat storage, particularly around the abdomen.

Additionally, alcohol's impact on blood pressure and lipid profiles cannot be overlooked. Alcohol raises triglyceride levels, a type of fat in the blood, and lowers levels of high-density lipoprotein (HDL), or "good cholesterol." High triglycerides and low HDL are hallmarks of metabolic syndrome. Combined with alcohol-induced insulin resistance, these factors create a perfect storm for metabolic health decline.

Weight gain is another significant concern tied to alcohol consumption. Alcohol contains "empty calories," meaning it provides energy without any essential nutrients. A standard drink contains approximately 100–150 calories, but sugary mixers or specialty cocktails can push that number even higher. These extra calories can contribute to weight gain, particularly when consumed frequently.

When insulin resistance is present, the body struggles to utilize glucose for energy, turning to fat storage instead. Alcohol also suppresses fat oxidation, the process by which the body burns fat for fuel. This dual effect—impairing fat burning while encouraging fat storage—explains why regular alcohol consumption is often linked to weight gain and obesity.

Furthermore, alcohol can influence appetite and food choices. Studies have shown that alcohol consumption increases cravings for high-calorie, carbohydrate-rich foods. This is partly due to its effect on the brain's reward system, which becomes more sensitive to the pleasure derived from eating. Over time, these poor dietary choices can compound the weight gain caused by alcohol's direct metabolic effects.

By adopting healthier drinking patterns, making informed dietary choices, and staying physically active, you can protect your metabolic health and reduce your risk of chronic diseases. Ultimately, moderation and mindfulness are the keys to enjoying alcohol responsibly while prioritizing your long-term well-being.

Microbial Toxins and the Brain

Case Study #15: Toxins from gut bacteria such as lipopolysaccharides (LPS) increase in the bloodstream after alcohol consumption, reaching the brain and contributing to neurodegenerative changes.

One significant consequence of alcohol consumption is its ability to disturb the gut microbiome, leading to an increase in the bloodstream of harmful substances such as **lipopolysaccharides** (LPS). These toxins, originating from gut bacteria, can reach the brain and contribute to neurodegenerative changes.

Lipopolysaccharides are large molecules found on the outer membrane of Gram-negative bacteria in the gut. These substances play a structural role in bacteria but can become highly toxic to humans when they enter the bloodstream. Under normal circumstances, the intestinal lining forms a strong barrier that prevents LPS from escaping the gut. However, alcohol consumption disrupts this delicate barrier, a condition known as "leaky gut."

When alcohol is consumed, it inflames and damages the gut lining, creating gaps that allow LPS and other toxins to pass through. This process, called intestinal permeability, facilitates the movement of harmful substances into the bloodstream, triggering systemic inflammation. Elevated levels of LPS in the bloodstream are known as endotoxemia, a condition linked to multiple health problems.

Once in the bloodstream, lipopolysaccharides do not remain confined to one area. Instead, they can travel throughout the body, including to the brain. The blood-brain barrier, which ordinarily serves as a defense mechanism to protect the brain from harmful substances, can also be compromised by alcohol consumption. This allows LPS to infiltrate the brain, where they wreak havoc on neurological health.

LPS activate immune responses both in the bloodstream and within the brain. In the brain, they stimulate the activity of microglia—immune cells responsible for clearing debris and protecting neural tissues. However, when overactivated, microglia release excessive inflammatory chemicals, contributing to neuroinflammation. Chronic neuroinflammation has been strongly linked to neurodegenerative diseases, including Alzheimer's disease and Parkinson's disease.

Additionally, LPS-induced neuroinflammation can disrupt the balance of neurotransmitters and impair brain function, leading to symptoms such as brain fog, anxiety, depression, and memory issues. These symptoms often go unnoticed or are attributed to other factors, masking the underlying connection between gut health, alcohol consumption, and brain health.

Systemic Effects of Elevated LPS Levels: More Than Just Brain Health

The impact of LPS in the bloodstream extends far beyond the brain. Endotoxemia triggers systemic inflammation, which is a major contributor to chronic diseases. Here are some of the key systems affected:

Liver Health: The liver bears the brunt of LPS-induced damage due to its role in detoxifying harmful substances. Alcohol consumption already places significant stress on the liver, leading to conditions like fatty liver disease, hepatitis, and cirrhosis. When combined with LPS, the inflammatory response is amplified, accelerating liver damage and impairing its ability to filter toxins effectively.

Cardiovascular System: Chronic inflammation caused by elevated LPS levels can lead to endothelial dysfunction, a precursor to cardiovascular diseases. It can increase the risk of atherosclerosis (plaque buildup in arteries), high blood pressure, and other heart-related conditions.

Immune System: Persistent exposure to LPS can lead to immune system dysregulation. While it may trigger excessive inflammation in some areas, it can also suppress immune responses in others, leaving the body vulnerable to infections and reducing its ability to fight off pathogens.

Metabolic Health: LPS-induced inflammation interferes with insulin signaling, contributing to insulin resistance and increasing the risk of type 2 diabetes. It also disrupts metabolic pathways, potentially leading to weight gain and difficulty maintaining a healthy weight.

Alcohol's Impact on the Gut Microbiome: The Root Cause

The gut microbiome, composed of trillions of bacteria, fungi, and other microorganisms, plays a crucial role in maintaining overall health. Alcohol consumption disrupts the delicate balance of this ecosystem in several ways:

Reduction in Beneficial Bacteria Alcohol reduces the population of beneficial bacteria such as *Lactobacillus* and *Bifidobacterium*, which help maintain gut integrity and prevent harmful bacteria from flourishing.

Overgrowth of Harmful Bacteria Alcohol promotes the growth of Gram-negative bacteria that produce lipopolysaccharides. This creates an imbalance, known as dysbiosis, which exacerbates gut permeability and inflammation.

Altered Metabolism Alcohol disrupts the metabolic activity of gut bacteria, further contributing to the production of harmful substances and reducing the production of beneficial metabolites like short-chain fatty acids (SCFAs).

The cumulative effects of these changes weaken the gut's defenses, making it easier for LPS to escape into the bloodstream and wreak havoc throughout the body.

Understanding the connection between alcohol, gut health, and neurodegenerative changes underscores the importance of adopting strategies to minimize these harmful effects. Here are some practical steps:

Limit Alcohol Consumption Reducing or eliminating alcohol intake is the most effective way to protect gut and brain health. For those who choose to drink, moderation is key. Guidelines recommend no more than one drink per day for women and two drinks per day for men.

Support Gut Barrier Integrity Consuming a diet rich in nutrients that support gut health can help repair the intestinal lining. Key nutrients include:

Glutamine An amino acid that helps rebuild the gut lining.

Zinc A mineral essential for maintaining gut barrier function.

Omega-3 Fatty Acids Anti-inflammatory compounds that support gut health.

Promote a Balanced Microbiome with probiotics and prebiotics.

Probiotics These beneficial bacteria can help restore balance to the gut microbiome and reduce inflammation. Fermented foods like yogurt, kefir, and sauerkraut are excellent sources.

Prebiotics Non-digestible fibers found in foods like garlic, onions, and bananas feed beneficial gut bacteria, promoting their growth.

Combat Inflammation Incorporating anti-inflammatory foods, such as turmeric, ginger, and leafy greens, can help counteract the effects of LPS and reduce systemic inflammation.

Stay Hydrated Adequate hydration supports liver function and helps flush out toxins more efficiently, reducing the burden of LPS on the body.

Regular Physical Activity Exercise has been shown to improve gut microbiota composition, reduce inflammation, and enhance overall health, providing a protective effect against LPS-induced damage.

The Bigger Picture: Why This Matters

The relationship between alcohol consumption, gut health, and brain function highlights the interconnectedness of the body's systems. Toxins from gut bacteria, such as lipopolysaccharides, serve as a stark reminder of how lifestyle choices can have far-reaching consequences on physical and mental health. By understanding these connections, individuals can make informed decisions to protect their health and reduce the risk of chronic diseases.

While occasional alcohol consumption may seem harmless, the science behind its impact on the gut and brain suggests otherwise. For those seeking to optimize their health, minimizing alcohol intake and supporting the gut microbiome through diet and lifestyle changes is a powerful step toward a healthier, more resilient body and mind.

Suppression of Probiotics

Case Study #16: Alcohol consumption suppresses beneficial bacteria like *Bifidobacterium*, which are crucial for maintaining gut integrity and reducing inflammation.

One of the most significant effects of alcohol is its suppression of beneficial bacteria, particularly *Bifidobacterium*. These microbes play a crucial role in maintaining gut integrity and reducing inflammation.

Bifidobacterium is a genus of bacteria that is naturally present in the human gastrointestinal tract. These microbes are classified as probiotics, meaning they provide health benefits when present in adequate amounts. Bifidobacterium contributes to numerous vital processes in the body:

Maintaining Gut Integrity These bacteria help strengthen the intestinal lining by promoting the production of mucus, a barrier that prevents harmful pathogens and toxins from entering the bloodstream.

Reducing Inflammation Bifidobacterium modulates the immune system and decreases inflammation by producing short-chain fatty acids (SCFAs), such as butyrate. SCFAs nourish colon cells and reduce inflammatory responses in the gut and throughout the body.

Balancing the Gut Microbiome Bifidobacterium suppresses the growth of harmful bacteria by producing lactic acid and other antimicrobial substances, keeping the gut microbiome balanced and healthy.

A well-functioning gut microbiome, with an adequate population of Bifidobacterium, supports digestion, nutrient absorption, and mental health. Unfortunately, alcohol consumption can severely disrupt this balance.

Alcohol's toxic effects extend beyond the liver and brain; it wreaks havoc on the gut microbiome. Ethanol, the primary active ingredient in alcoholic beverages, acts as a *broad-spectrum antimicrobial agent.* While this may sound beneficial at first, it's problematic because it kills both harmful and beneficial bacteria indiscriminately. Bifidobacterium, being particularly sensitive to ethanol, experiences a sharp decline in populations when alcohol is consumed.

Damage to the Gut Lining

A reduction in Bifidobacterium compromises the integrity of the gut lining. Without sufficient levels of these beneficial bacteria, the protective mucus layer thins, making the gut more permeable. This condition, commonly known as "leaky gut syndrome," allows toxins, undigested food particles, and harmful bacteria to pass into the bloodstream. Leaky gut can trigger widespread inflammation, contributing to chronic conditions such as autoimmune diseases, metabolic syndrome, and even mental health disorders like anxiety and depression.

By suppressing Bifidobacterium, alcohol indirectly increases inflammation throughout the body. The loss of SCFA production, particularly butyrate, removes a key anti-inflammatory mechanism. This leaves the gut and the body vulnerable to the damaging effects of pro-inflammatory molecules. Chronic inflammation is a precursor to many health issues, including heart disease, diabetes, and certain types of cancer.

When alcohol disrupts the balance of beneficial bacteria like Bifidobacterium, the consequences extend far beyond the gut.

The gut microbiome is essential for breaking down complex carbohydrates and producing essential vitamins like B12 and K2.

With fewer Bifidobacterium present, digestive efficiency decreases. Symptoms such as bloating, constipation, and diarrhea become more common. Moreover, the reduced production of SCFAs impairs colon health, increasing the risk of colorectal diseases.

Additionally, approximately 70% of the immune system resides in the gut, heavily reliant on signals from beneficial bacteria like Bifidobacterium. A weakened population of these bacteria compromises the gut-associated lymphoid tissue (GALT), diminishing the body's ability to fight infections and increasing susceptibility to illnesses.

The gut-brain axis, a bidirectional communication system between the gut and brain, relies heavily on a healthy microbiome. *Bifidobacterium influences the production of neurotransmitters such as serotonin,* often referred to as the "feel-good" hormone. Alcohol-induced suppression of Bifidobacterium can lead to imbalances in neurotransmitter production, contributing to mood disorders, including depression and anxiety.

An imbalanced gut microbiome, skewed by alcohol consumption, affects metabolism and weight regulation. Harmful bacteria thrive in the absence of beneficial microbes, promoting cravings for sugar and refined carbohydrates. This creates a cycle of poor eating habits and weight gain, exacerbated by alcohol's empty calories.

The relationship between alcohol and gut health underscores the importance of making informed choices to support a balanced microbiome. Bifidobacterium is a cornerstone of gut integrity and overall wellness, and its suppression by alcohol can have far-reaching consequences. By understanding the role these beneficial bacteria play and taking proactive steps to protect them, you can safeguard your health for years to come. Reducing alcohol intake, eating a balanced diet, and incorporating healthy lifestyle habits are powerful strategies for promoting gut health and living a healthier, more vibrant life.

Oxidative Stress in the Gut

Case Study #17: Alcohol increases oxidative stress in the gut lining, damaging cells and further weakening the intestinal barrier. This oxidative damage perpetuates gut-brain axis dysfunction.

Alcohol consumption has profound effects on the body, particularly the gastrointestinal system. One of the most significant ways alcohol influences gut health is through oxidative stress—a harmful imbalance between free radicals and antioxidants in the body. Oxidative stress induced by alcohol consumption directly damages the gut lining, impairing its essential functions and contributing to systemic health issues.

The gut lining serves as a critical barrier, preventing harmful substances from entering the bloodstream while allowing nutrients to be absorbed. When alcohol is consumed, it increases the production of reactive oxygen species (ROS), leading to oxidative damage. These reactive molecules attack the cells of the intestinal lining, breaking down tight junctions—the protein structures that hold the cells of the gut barrier together. This weakening of the intestinal barrier is often referred to as "leaky gut" and is a precursor to a host of health problems, including inflammation and gut-brain axis dysfunction.

When alcohol enters the digestive system, it undergoes metabolism primarily in the liver, but significant processes also occur in the gut. *During alcohol metabolism, enzymes such as alcohol dehydrogenase (ADH) and cytochrome P450 (CYP2E1) produce byproducts, including acetaldehyde and free radicals.* Acetaldehyde, a highly toxic compound, is a major contributor to oxidative stress in the gut lining.

Excessive alcohol consumption overwhelms the body's natural antioxidant defenses, such as glutathione and superoxide dismutase, leading to the accumulation of free radicals. These molecules attack the lipid membranes of gut cells, causing lipid peroxidation—a process that destabilizes cell membranes and leads to cell death. As gut cells die or become dysfunctional, the integrity of the intestinal barrier is compromised, allowing harmful substances like bacteria, toxins, and undigested food particles to enter the bloodstream. This condition—known as intestinal permeability—is a key factor in systemic inflammation and chronic diseases.

The gut and brain are in constant communication through a complex network called the gut-brain axis. This bi-directional communication system relies on neural, hormonal, and immunological signals to maintain homeostasis. When oxidative stress damages the gut lining, it disrupts this delicate communication system in several ways.

First, increased intestinal permeability caused by alcohol-induced oxidative damage allows harmful substances to enter the bloodstream. These substances can trigger an immune response, leading to the release of pro-inflammatory cytokines. These inflammatory molecules can cross the blood-brain barrier, contributing to neuroinflammation and impairing brain function. This cascade of events perpetuates a cycle of gut-brain axis dysfunction.

Second, alcohol's impact on the gut microbiome exacerbates this dysfunction. Alcohol consumption alters the balance of gut bacteria, reducing beneficial strains like Lactobacillus and Bifidobacterium while promoting the growth of harmful bacteria. This microbial imbalance, or dysbiosis, produces additional toxins that further damage the gut lining and influence the brain's signaling pathways. *Dysbiosis is closely linked to mood disorders, cognitive impairment, and cravings, perpetuating alcohol dependency.*

The oxidative stress and inflammation caused by alcohol consumption extend beyond the gut, contributing to a range of chronic diseases. For instance, the pro-inflammatory state triggered by a compromised gut barrier has been linked to cardiovascular disease, liver disease, and metabolic disorders such as type 2 diabetes. The connection between gut health and systemic inflammation underscores the importance of maintaining intestinal integrity.

Alcohol-induced oxidative damage also has a direct impact on the immune system. The immune cells located in the gut, known as gut-associated lymphoid tissue (GALT), play a crucial role in defending the body against pathogens. When oxidative stress damages the gut lining, it weakens GALT, leaving the body more susceptible to infections and illnesses. This weakened immune response is particularly concerning for individuals who consume alcohol regularly, as their bodies may struggle to fight off even minor infections.

Alcohol's impact on the gut and gut-brain axis underscores the importance of maintaining a healthy intestinal barrier. Oxidative stress induced by alcohol consumption damages gut cells, weakens the intestinal barrier, and disrupts the gut-brain communication system, perpetuating a cycle of inflammation and dysfunction. However, these effects are not irreversible. By reducing alcohol intake, supporting antioxidant defenses, and promoting gut health, individuals can repair damage, restore balance, and improve overall health. Understanding the intricate relationship between the gut and brain empowers individuals to make informed choices for a healthier, more resilient body and mind.

Alcohol and Mood Disorders

Case Study #18: A disrupted microbiome has been linked to depression and anxiety. Alcohol's impact on the gut-brain axis exacerbates these conditions, as shown in a study published in *Psychiatry Research*.

The human gut and brain share a remarkable and intricate connection that researchers are only beginning to fully understand. This relationship, known as the gut-brain axis, is a two-way communication system that links the central nervous system (CNS) with the enteric nervous system (ENS) in the gastrointestinal tract. Through this connection, the gut microbiome—the collection of trillions of microorganisms residing in the digestive system—plays a critical role in influencing mental health.

The gut microbiome communicates with the brain via multiple pathways, including the vagus nerve, immune signaling, and the production of neurotransmitters like serotonin, dopamine, and gamma-aminobutyric acid (GABA). *Remarkably, the gut produces up to 90% of the body's serotonin,* a key neurotransmitter that helps regulate mood, appetite, and sleep. When the delicate balance of the gut microbiome is disrupted, the effects can ripple through the body, potentially leading to mental health disorders such as depression and anxiety.

Alcohol consumption has a profound and often detrimental effect on the gut microbiome. Even moderate drinking can disrupt the balance of beneficial bacteria in the gut, allowing harmful bacteria to proliferate. Chronic alcohol use exacerbates this imbalance, causing inflammation in the gut lining, a condition known as "leaky gut syndrome."

Leaky gut syndrome occurs when the intestinal lining becomes permeable, allowing toxins, bacteria, and undigested food particles to pass into the bloodstream. This triggers an immune response and chronic inflammation, which can further impair the gut's ability to function. Studies have shown that alcohol-induced gut dysbiosis leads to a reduction in microbial diversity, which is a hallmark of a healthy microbiome. When diversity diminishes, the gut's ability to produce essential neurotransmitters and regulate the immune system weakens, contributing to mental health challenges.

This study published in *Psychiatry Research* underscores the link between alcohol's impact on the gut and mental health conditions like depression and anxiety. The research highlights how alcohol-induced disruptions in the gut microbiome can affect the gut-brain axis, exacerbating symptoms of these disorders. For example, a disrupted gut microbiome may reduce the production of serotonin, contributing to feelings of sadness, fatigue, and hopelessness commonly associated with depression.

Anxiety, too, has been linked to gut health. Harmful bacteria in the gut can produce metabolites that interfere with the brain's signaling pathways, heightening feelings of worry and fear. Moreover, chronic inflammation caused by a leaky gut may increase the risk of neuroinflammation, a condition associated with both depression and anxiety. Alcohol's role in amplifying these conditions cannot be overstated, as its effects on the gut-brain axis create a cycle of worsening mental health and continued microbiome disruption.

One of the lesser-known effects of alcohol on the gut-brain axis is its ability to fuel cravings for more alcohol. This phenomenon occurs because harmful bacteria in a disrupted microbiome can influence the brain's reward system. Certain gut bacteria thrive on sugar and alcohol, producing chemicals that signal the brain to crave these substances.

This feedback loop not only perpetuates excessive alcohol consumption but also deepens the cycle of gut dysbiosis and mental health decline. For individuals struggling with depression or anxiety, these cravings can feel nearly impossible to resist, leading to a downward spiral that is difficult to break without targeted interventions. Addressing the root cause—gut health—is therefore essential for long-term recovery and improved mental well-being.

Altered Gut Hormones

Alcohol consumption can have far-reaching effects on the body, particularly on the gut and its crucial role in regulating hunger and satiety. Two key hormones, ghrelin and leptin, are responsible for managing how the body perceives hunger and fullness. Ghrelin, often referred to as the "hunger hormone," stimulates appetite, while leptin, the "satiety hormone," signals to the brain that the body has had enough to eat. When alcohol is introduced into the system, it disrupts the delicate balance between these two hormones, often leading to increased appetite and poor dietary choices.

Ghrelin: The Hunger Hormone on Overdrive

Ghrelin is produced primarily in the stomach and plays a pivotal role in signaling hunger to the brain. Normally, ghrelin levels rise before meals, prompting you to eat, and fall after meals, signaling satiety.

However, alcohol consumption has been shown to increase ghrelin levels, even when caloric needs have already been met. This increase can create a sensation of excessive hunger, leading individuals to eat more than they would otherwise.

Studies have demonstrated that alcohol not only elevates ghrelin levels but also makes the body more sensitive to the hormone's effects. This means that even a small rise in ghrelin caused by alcohol can have a disproportionately large impact on hunger cues. The result is a phenomenon known as "hyperphagia" or abnormally increased food consumption, often characterized by cravings for high-calorie, high-fat, and sugary foods. These cravings can contribute to weight gain, especially if alcohol consumption becomes a regular habit.

Leptin: The Silenced Satiety Hormone

While ghrelin encourages hunger, leptin acts as a counterbalance by promoting satiety. Leptin is produced by fat cells and communicates with the hypothalamus in the brain to regulate food intake and energy expenditure. When you've eaten enough, leptin levels rise, signaling to your brain that it's time to stop eating. Unfortunately, alcohol disrupts this process as well.

Research has shown that alcohol consumption can suppress leptin production, effectively silencing the body's natural "stop" signal. This suppression can make it harder to recognize when you're full, leading to overeating. Moreover, chronic alcohol use has been linked to leptin resistance, a condition in which the brain no longer responds appropriately to leptin signals. This can create a vicious cycle of overeating and weight gain, as the body struggles to regulate food intake effectively.

The disruption of ghrelin and leptin by alcohol doesn't just increase appetite—it also alters the types of foods you're likely to crave. Alcohol has a unique ability to lower inhibitions and impair decision-making, which extends to dietary choices. Combined with elevated ghrelin and suppressed leptin levels, this can lead to a preference for calorie-dense, nutrient-poor foods.

Studies have shown that people who drink alcohol tend to consume more fried foods, sweets, and other unhealthy options compared to those who abstain. The combination of alcohol's effect on hunger hormones and its impact on the brain's reward system can make high-fat, sugary foods particularly appealing. These foods provide a quick energy boost, which may temporarily counteract the lethargy and low blood sugar often caused by alcohol, but they also contribute to long-term health issues like obesity, diabetes, and cardiovascular disease.

The short-term effects of alcohol on hunger hormones can lead to immediate overeating, but the long-term consequences are even more concerning. Regular alcohol consumption can contribute to chronic hormonal imbalances that affect overall metabolism and body composition.

For instance, persistent elevation of ghrelin levels can lead to habitual overeating, while chronic suppression of leptin can make it increasingly difficult to recognize and respond to satiety cues.

These hormonal disruptions also have a ripple effect on other aspects of health. Increased body weight and fat accumulation, particularly around the abdomen, are common outcomes of alcohol-induced hormonal imbalance. This type of fat, known as visceral fat, is especially dangerous because it's associated with a higher risk of metabolic syndrome, type 2 diabetes, and cardiovascular disease. Additionally, leptin resistance can exacerbate these conditions, as the body becomes less capable of regulating energy balance and blood sugar levels effectively.

Alcohol's impact on hunger hormones like ghrelin and leptin is just one example of how lifestyle choices can affect the body's intricate hormonal systems. By understanding these mechanisms and taking proactive steps to support hormonal balance, you can make more informed decisions about alcohol consumption and its role in your overall health.

Ultimately, maintaining a healthy relationship with food and alcohol requires a holistic approach that prioritizes balanced nutrition, regular exercise, and mindful habits. While occasional indulgence is unlikely to cause significant harm, being aware of alcohol's effects on hunger and dietary choices can empower you to make choices that support long-term health and well-being.

Immune System Suppression

Case Study #20: A study in *Immunology Today* found that alcohol disrupts gut microbes that support the immune system, making the body more susceptible to infections.

Alcohol consumption has a profound impact on the gut microbiome, disrupting the delicate balance of microbes that play a crucial role in supporting the immune system. This disruption leaves the body more vulnerable to infections, highlighting a lesser-known but vital aspect of alcohol's effects on overall health. Understanding the link between alcohol, the gut, and immunity can empower individuals to make more informed decisions about their alcohol consumption and prioritize their health.

The gut microbiome consists of trillions of bacteria, fungi, and other microorganisms that live in the digestive tract. These microbes are not merely passive residents; they actively contribute to numerous bodily functions, including digestion, nutrient absorption, and immune system regulation. Approximately 70% of the body's immune cells are found in the gut, underscoring the central role of this organ in protecting the body from harmful pathogens.

Beneficial gut bacteria, such as *Lactobacillus* and *Bifidobacterium*, produce metabolites like short-chain fatty acids (SCFAs) that help regulate immune responses. These metabolites maintain the integrity of the gut lining, preventing harmful substances from entering the bloodstream and triggering systemic inflammation. When the gut microbiome is balanced, it creates a robust defense system that helps fend off infections and promotes overall well-being.

Alcohol disrupts this delicate ecosystem in several ways. First, it alters the composition of the gut microbiome by reducing the population of beneficial bacteria and promoting the growth of harmful bacteria. Research shows that chronic alcohol consumption can lead to an overgrowth of pathogens like *Escherichia coli* and *Clostridium difficile*, which can compromise gut health and the immune system.

Second, alcohol increases gut permeability, a condition often referred to as "leaky gut." The intestinal lining acts as a barrier, preventing toxins and undigested food particles from entering the bloodstream. When alcohol damages this barrier, it allows these harmful substances to pass through, triggering an immune response and systemic inflammation. This inflammatory state can weaken the body's ability to fight off infections and contribute to the development of chronic diseases.

Third, alcohol consumption can suppress the production of SCFAs and other essential metabolites, disrupting the immune-modulating functions of the gut microbiome. Without these critical compounds, the immune system's ability to respond to threats is significantly impaired.

Increased Susceptibility to Infections

The disruption of the gut microbiome caused by alcohol makes the body more susceptible to infections. When the balance of gut bacteria is disturbed, the immune system struggles to respond effectively to harmful pathogens. For instance, studies have found that individuals who consume alcohol excessively are more prone to respiratory infections, urinary tract infections, and gastrointestinal illnesses.

Additionally, alcohol's impact on gut permeability allows harmful bacteria and their byproducts, such as lipopolysaccharides (LPS), to enter the bloodstream. LPS are known to trigger strong inflammatory responses, which can overwhelm the immune system and increase the risk of sepsis, a potentially life-threatening condition. The combination of a weakened immune system and increased systemic inflammation creates a perfect storm for infections to take hold and spread.

The effects of alcohol on the gut microbiome and immune system are not limited to short-term risks. Chronic alcohol consumption can lead to long-lasting changes in gut health, making it harder for the microbiome to recover even after alcohol use is reduced or stopped. These persistent imbalances can contribute to a range of health issues, including:

Chronic Inflammation Continuous immune activation due to a leaky gut can result in chronic inflammation, which is a precursor to many diseases, including cardiovascular disease, diabetes, and autoimmune disorders.

Nutrient Deficiencies A disrupted gut microbiome can impair nutrient absorption, leading to deficiencies in vitamins and minerals essential for immune function, such as vitamin D, zinc, and magnesium.

Mental Health Challenges The gut-brain axis, a bidirectional communication network between the gut and the brain, can be affected by alcohol-induced gut microbiome disruption. This can contribute to anxiety, depression, and other mental health conditions.

Liver Disease Alcohol-related liver diseases, such as fatty liver, hepatitis, and cirrhosis, are closely linked to gut microbiome imbalances and systemic inflammation.

Fortunately, there are ways to mitigate the impact of alcohol on the gut microbiome and support immune health. Adopting a gut-friendly lifestyle can help restore balance and promote resilience against infections. Reducing alcohol intake or abstaining altogether is the most effective way to protect the gut microbiome and immune system. Consuming a variety of fruits, vegetables, whole grains, and fermented foods can promote the growth of beneficial gut bacteria. Foods rich in prebiotics, such as garlic, onions, and bananas, provide fuel for these microbes. Probiotic supplements and foods like yogurt, kefir, and sauerkraut can help replenish beneficial bacteria and restore gut balance. Drinking plenty of water supports digestion and helps flush toxins from the body, reducing the burden on the gut and liver. Quality sleep and stress-reduction practices, such as mindfulness or yoga, can support a healthy gut-brain axis and improve overall immune function.

The study in *Immunology Today* underscores a critical but often overlooked aspect of alcohol's impact on health. By disrupting the gut microbiome, alcohol compromises the immune system and increases vulnerability to infections. Recognizing this connection can motivate individuals to prioritize their gut health and consider the broader implications of their drinking habits.

Taking proactive steps to support the gut microbiome—through dietary changes, reduced alcohol consumption, and stress management—can strengthen immunity and promote long-term health. As research continues to uncover the intricate relationship between the gut and the immune system, one thing remains clear: a healthy gut is the foundation of a resilient and thriving body.

Impaired Cognitive Function

Case Study #21: Alcohol's disruption of the gut-brain connection has been linked to impaired cognitive function, including slower reaction times and reduced memory retention.

Alcohol consumption has long been associated with short-term euphoria and relaxation, but its effects on the body go much deeper, particularly when it comes to the gut-brain connection. Recent studies have shown that alcohol can significantly disrupt this vital communication network, leading to impaired cognitive functions such as slower reaction times and reduced memory retention. To understand the full scope of alcohol's influence, it's essential to delve into the mechanisms at play between the gut and the brain and explore how these disruptions affect overall health and mental clarity.

The gut and brain are closely linked through a complex communication system known as the gut-brain axis. This system relies on chemical and physical connections, including the vagus nerve, a direct line of communication between the gut and brain, and signaling molecules like neurotransmitters and hormones.

Within this axis, the gut microbiome—composed of trillions of bacteria, fungi, and other microbes—plays a critical role in maintaining balance.

A healthy gut microbiome supports the production of neurotransmitters like serotonin and dopamine, which influence mood, memory, and reaction times. Conversely, an imbalanced microbiome can lead to the release of harmful substances, which can cross the gut lining and affect the brain. Alcohol, unfortunately, is a major disruptor of this balance, introducing a cascade of problems that impair the gut-brain connection.

Alcohol consumption can lead to dysbiosis, a state of imbalance in the gut microbiome where harmful bacteria outnumber beneficial ones. This imbalance compromises the gut lining, increasing its permeability—a condition often referred to as "leaky gut." When the gut lining is compromised, toxins, bacteria, and inflammatory molecules can escape into the bloodstream, eventually reaching the brain.

Leaky gut syndrome caused by alcohol has profound implications for the brain. Inflammatory molecules released due to dysbiosis can pass through the blood-brain barrier, a protective shield meant to keep harmful substances away from the brain. Once inside, these inflammatory agents can interfere with neurotransmitter production and signaling, which are essential for cognitive processes like memory and reaction time.

Cognitive Impairments Linked to Alcohol's Disruption of the Gut-Brain Connection

The inflammation and disruption caused by alcohol don't just harm the gut; they also significantly impact brain function. One of the most noticeable cognitive effects of alcohol is slower reaction times. This occurs because alcohol hampers the ability of neurotransmitters to send and receive signals efficiently. For example, the neurotransmitter glutamate, which plays a critical role in learning and memory, is particularly vulnerable to the effects of alcohol-induced inflammation.

Additionally, alcohol consumption impairs memory retention. Studies have shown that the inflammatory response triggered by alcohol reduces the hippocampus's ability to process and store new information. The hippocampus, a critical brain region for memory formation, relies on healthy neural pathways and neurotransmitter activity. When these are compromised by alcohol-related inflammation, short-term and long-term memory are affected, leading to forgetfulness and difficulty concentrating.

Long-Term Effects: Chronic Cognitive Decline and Neurodegeneration

While occasional drinking may cause temporary disruptions in the gut-brain connection, chronic alcohol consumption can lead to long-term cognitive decline. Persistent inflammation in the brain contributes to the degeneration of neurons, which are responsible for transmitting information throughout the nervous system. Over time, this can increase the risk of developing neurodegenerative diseases such as Alzheimer's and Parkinson's.

Alcohol-related gut microbiome imbalances are also linked to mental health disorders like anxiety and depression. Because the gut produces about 90% of the body's serotonin—a neurotransmitter often called the "happy chemical"—a disrupted microbiome can significantly impact mood regulation. Chronic alcohol consumption exacerbates this effect, creating a cycle where poor mental health leads to more drinking, further damaging the gut-brain axis.

Dopamine Dysregulation

Case Study #22: The microbiome influences dopamine production. Alcohol disrupts these pathways, leading to mood instability and increased cravings.

The human gut is often referred to as the "second brain," and for good reason. Within the gut resides a complex ecosystem of microorganisms known as the microbiome, which plays a pivotal role in maintaining overall health. Among its many functions, the microbiome directly impacts the production and regulation of dopamine—a neurotransmitter responsible for feelings of pleasure, motivation, and reward. A healthy microbiome contributes to balanced dopamine levels, supporting mood stability and reducing cravings for harmful substances. However, when the microbiome becomes disrupted, the effects on dopamine production can lead to significant consequences for mental and physical health.

Dopamine production involves a fascinating interplay between the gut and the brain. Specific gut bacteria synthesize precursors to dopamine, such as tyrosine and phenylalanine, which are then transported to the brain to facilitate neurotransmitter production.

Additionally, the vagus nerve—a crucial communication pathway between the gut and the brain—helps relay signals about gut health and activity. When the microbiome is balanced, this system functions efficiently, promoting not only healthy dopamine levels but also improved emotional well-being and reduced susceptibility to addictive behaviors.

Alcohol consumption is a significant disruptor of the gut-brain axis, particularly its impact on dopamine production. Initially, drinking alcohol releases a flood of dopamine in the brain, creating feelings of euphoria and relaxation. This surge in dopamine reinforces the behavior, encouraging individuals to drink more. However, over time, chronic alcohol use leads to a depletion of dopamine and damages the gut microbiome, creating a vicious cycle of dependency and mood instability.

Alcohol disrupts the microbiome by killing beneficial bacteria and promoting the overgrowth of harmful strains. This imbalance, known as dysbiosis, interferes with the gut's ability to produce dopamine precursors effectively. Additionally, the inflammation caused by alcohol damages the gut lining, increasing intestinal permeability, or "leaky gut syndrome." This condition allows toxins and bacteria to enter the bloodstream, further exacerbating inflammation and impairing communication between the gut and the brain.

The result is a two-fold problem: reduced dopamine production in the gut and impaired signaling to the brain. Individuals may experience mood swings, anxiety, and depression as their bodies struggle to maintain normal dopamine levels. Furthermore, *the brain's reward system becomes desensitized to natural sources of pleasure,* driving increased cravings for alcohol and other addictive substances as a means to artificially boost dopamine levels.

Mood Instability and Cravings: The Domino Effect

One of the most significant consequences of alcohol's disruption of the microbiome is its impact on mood stability. Dopamine plays a central role in regulating emotions, and when its production is compromised, individuals are more likely to experience *mood swings, irritability, and even symptoms of depression.* This emotional instability often perpetuates a cycle of alcohol use, as individuals turn to drinking in an attempt to self-medicate and alleviate their symptoms.

Cravings are another hallmark of disrupted dopamine pathways. When the gut microbiome is imbalanced, it can trigger powerful urges for alcohol and sugary foods. Harmful gut bacteria, which thrive on sugar and alcohol, *release chemical signals that influence the brain's reward centers, intensifying cravings.* This phenomenon highlights the profound connection between gut health and behavior, as the microbiome's state can directly influence an individual's choices and habits.

Restoring Gut Health to Support Dopamine Balance

The good news is that the gut microbiome is remarkably resilient, and steps can be taken to restore its balance and support healthy dopamine production. Addressing the damage caused by alcohol involves a combination of dietary changes, probiotic supplementation, and lifestyle adjustments.

A diet rich in fiber, prebiotics, and fermented foods can help rebuild the gut microbiome. Foods such as leafy greens, bananas, garlic, onions, and whole grains provide essential nutrients for beneficial bacteria. Fermented foods like yogurt, kefir, sauerkraut, and kimchi introduce live cultures that replenish the microbiome. Avoiding processed foods, excessive sugar, and alcohol is also crucial to preventing further damage.

Probiotic supplements can play a significant role in restoring gut health. Specific strains, such as *Lactobacillus rhamnosus* and

Bifidobacterium longum, have been shown to improve mood and support dopamine production. Additionally, supplements like L-tyrosine—a precursor to dopamine—can aid in replenishing neurotransmitter levels.

Incorporating regular exercise, practicing mindfulness, and reducing stress can also positively impact the gut-brain axis. Physical activity has been shown to increase dopamine levels, while stress management techniques help reduce inflammation and support overall gut health. Prioritizing adequate sleep is another critical factor, as restorative sleep allows the body to repair and maintain its systems, including the gut and brain.

The Long-Term Benefits of a Balanced Microbiome

Restoring and maintaining a healthy microbiome offers far-reaching benefits beyond dopamine production. A balanced microbiome supports immune function, reduces inflammation, and enhances overall well-being. Individuals who take proactive steps to improve their gut health often report increased energy, better focus, and a more stable mood. Perhaps most importantly, breaking the cycle of alcohol dependency and cravings becomes more achievable when the gut-brain axis is functioning optimally.

The connection between the microbiome and dopamine production underscores the profound influence of gut health on mental and emotional well-being. Alcohol's disruptive effects on this delicate system highlight the importance of addressing gut health in the context of addiction and recovery. By prioritizing a balanced microbiome through dietary and lifestyle changes, individuals can support healthy dopamine levels, reduce cravings, and foster long-term resilience against the challenges of modern life.

Reduction in SCFA Production

Case Study #23: Short-chain fatty acids (SCFAs) like butyrate are critical for gut and brain health. Alcohol reduces SCFA production, impairing gut integrity and brain function.

Short-chain fatty acids (SCFAs), including butyrate, acetate, and propionate, are key metabolites produced when gut bacteria ferment dietary fiber. These compounds play a crucial role in maintaining gut integrity, regulating inflammation, and supporting brain health. Among SCFAs, butyrate stands out for its profound effects on both the gut and brain, acting as a primary energy source for colon cells and influencing neurological function through the gut-brain axis.

Understanding the relationship between SCFAs, gut health, and brain health is essential for maintaining overall well-being. Yet, various lifestyle factors, including alcohol consumption, can disrupt the delicate balance of SCFAs in the gut, leading to significant health consequences.

SCFAs: The Unsung Heroes of Gut Health

The gut microbiome consists of trillions of microorganisms that work symbiotically with the human body to maintain health. SCFAs are among the most important byproducts of this partnership. When dietary fiber reaches the large intestine, gut bacteria ferment it, producing SCFAs in the process. These compounds have numerous benefits for gut health, including:

Maintaining Gut Barrier Integrity Butyrate serves as the primary energy source for colonocytes (cells lining the colon), promoting their growth and repair. This function helps to strengthen the intestinal barrier, preventing harmful substances like toxins and pathogens from entering the bloodstream.

Reducing Inflammation SCFAs modulate the immune system by influencing the activity of regulatory T cells, which help suppress excessive inflammation. This is crucial in preventing chronic conditions like inflammatory bowel disease (IBD).

Balancing Gut Microbiota The production of SCFAs fosters an environment conducive to the growth of beneficial bacteria, further enhancing gut health.

Without sufficient SCFA production, the gut barrier weakens, inflammation increases, and harmful bacteria may proliferate, setting the stage for various health issues.

The Gut-Brain Axis: Linking SCFAs to Brain Function

The gut and brain communicate through a complex network known as the gut-brain axis, which involves neural, hormonal, and immune pathways. SCFAs, particularly butyrate, play a pivotal role in this communication by:

Reducing Neuroinflammation Butyrate crosses the blood-brain barrier and exerts anti-inflammatory effects in the central nervous system. By reducing inflammation, it helps protect against neurodegenerative diseases like Alzheimer's and Parkinson's.

Promoting Brain-Derived Neurotrophic Factor (BDNF) Butyrate enhances the production of BDNF, a protein that supports the growth and survival of neurons. Higher levels of BDNF are associated with improved memory, learning, and overall cognitive function.

Regulating Mood and Behavior SCFAs influence the production of neurotransmitters like serotonin and dopamine, which are critical for mood regulation. A healthy gut microbiome with robust SCFA production can help reduce symptoms of anxiety and depression.

The connection between gut and brain health underscores the importance of maintaining optimal SCFA levels. Disruptions to SCFA production can impair gut function and lead to cognitive and emotional difficulties.

Alcohol consumption can severely disrupt the gut microbiome and reduce SCFA production, leading to a cascade of negative effects on both the gut and brain. Several mechanisms explain this disruption:

Impairing Gut Microbial Diversity Alcohol selectively promotes the growth of harmful bacteria while reducing the abundance of beneficial, fiber-fermenting bacteria. This imbalance, known as dysbiosis, results in lower SCFA production.

Weakening the Gut Barrier Reduced SCFA levels impair the integrity of the gut lining, making it more permeable. This condition, often referred to as "leaky gut," allows toxins and inflammatory substances to enter the bloodstream and reach the brain.

Increasing Inflammation Alcohol-induced reductions in SCFAs exacerbate inflammation in both the gut and brain. Chronic inflammation has been linked to conditions such as depression, anxiety, and cognitive decline.

Studies have shown that even moderate alcohol consumption can decrease butyrate levels significantly, highlighting the sensitivity of SCFA production to lifestyle factors. Over time, these disruptions can lead to chronic health problems that affect both physical and mental well-being.

Maintaining healthy SCFA levels requires a holistic approach that includes dietary and lifestyle changes. Here are key strategies to support SCFA production and counteract the negative effects of alcohol:

Increase Fiber Intake A diet rich in prebiotic fibers, such as those found in fruits, vegetables, legumes, and whole grains, provides the raw materials needed for SCFA production. Aim for at least 25-30 grams of fiber daily.

Incorporate Fermented Foods Foods like yogurt, kefir, sauerkraut, and kimchi contain probiotics that help maintain a healthy gut microbiome, enhancing SCFA production.

Limit Alcohol Consumption Reducing or eliminating alcohol intake allows the gut microbiome to recover and resume normal SCFA production. If quitting entirely is not feasible, consider moderating consumption to minimize its impact.

Consider Supplementation In some cases, supplements containing butyrate or prebiotics can help restore SCFA levels, particularly for individuals with gut dysbiosis or chronic inflammation.

Exercise Regularly Physical activity has been shown to promote microbial diversity and increase SCFA production. Aim for at least 150 minutes of moderate exercise per week.

Manage Stress Chronic stress can negatively impact the gut microbiome and reduce SCFA production. Practices like mindfulness meditation, yoga, and deep breathing can help mitigate these effects.

The Long-Term Consequences of Disrupted SCFA Production

A persistent reduction in SCFA production can have far-reaching consequences for both gut and brain health. Chronic gut inflammation and a weakened gut barrier may lead to systemic inflammation, increasing the risk of autoimmune diseases, metabolic disorders, and even certain cancers. Simultaneously, reduced SCFA levels can contribute to cognitive decline, mood disorders, and neurodegenerative diseases.

Understanding the importance of SCFAs highlights the need to prioritize gut health in daily life. While occasional alcohol consumption may not cause irreversible damage, chronic or excessive intake can significantly impair SCFA production and overall health. By making informed lifestyle choices, individuals can support their gut microbiome, enhance SCFA production, and promote lifelong well-being.

Short-chain fatty acids like butyrate are essential for maintaining the health of both the gut and brain. They support gut barrier integrity, regulate inflammation, and influence neurological function through the gut-brain axis. However, alcohol consumption can significantly reduce SCFA production, leading to a weakened gut barrier, increased inflammation, and impaired brain function.

By understanding the importance of SCFAs and adopting lifestyle changes that support their production, individuals can safeguard their gut and brain health. A balanced diet, regular exercise, and mindful habits are key to fostering a thriving gut microbiome and promoting overall well-being.

Increased Gut Permeability

Case Study #24: Alcohol increases gut permeability, allowing harmful microbes and toxins to enter the bloodstream, affecting brain function and overall health.

Gut permeability refers to the ability of the intestinal lining to act as a barrier, selectively allowing nutrients to pass into the bloodstream while keeping harmful substances, such as toxins, microbes, and undigested food particles, out. This protective mechanism is crucial for maintaining overall health and supporting the immune system. However, when this barrier becomes compromised—a condition often referred to as "leaky gut syndrome"—harmful substances can seep into the bloodstream, leading to inflammation and other systemic health issues.

Alcohol consumption has been shown to directly compromise gut permeability. The intestinal lining is composed of tight junctions, which are specialized proteins that seal the spaces between cells in the gut wall. Alcohol weakens these tight junctions, creating gaps that allow harmful microbes, toxins, and inflammatory molecules to pass into the bloodstream. This phenomenon, commonly known as "gut leakage," can lead to widespread inflammation throughout the body.

Moreover, alcohol increases the production of harmful bacterial byproducts, such as lipopolysaccharides (LPS), which can further damage the gut lining. When LPS enters the bloodstream, it triggers an immune response that may exacerbate inflammation and contribute to chronic health conditions, including liver disease, cardiovascular issues, and neurological disorders.

The gut microbiome—a diverse ecosystem of bacteria, fungi, and other microorganisms—plays a key role in maintaining gut health. A balanced microbiome supports digestion, produces essential vitamins, and protects against harmful pathogens. However, alcohol consumption disrupts this delicate balance by reducing beneficial bacteria and encouraging the growth of harmful strains.

This microbial imbalance, known as dysbiosis, can further weaken the gut barrier. Harmful bacteria produce toxins that erode the gut lining, compounding the effects of alcohol on gut permeability. Over time, this cycle of damage can lead to chronic inflammation and increase the risk of autoimmune diseases, food intolerances, and even mental health disorders.

When the gut barrier is compromised, the harmful substances that enter the bloodstream can have far-reaching effects on the body. Some of the most significant impacts include:

Brain Function and Mental Health The gut and brain are closely connected through the gut-brain axis, a bidirectional communication network involving the nervous system, immune system, and gut microbiota. Increased gut permeability allows toxins and inflammatory molecules to reach the brain, where they can disrupt neurotransmitter production and contribute to mood disorders, anxiety, and cognitive decline.

Immune System Dysregulation The immune system is highly active in the gut, constantly monitoring for harmful invaders. When the gut barrier is compromised, the immune system becomes overstimulated, leading to chronic inflammation. Over time, this can weaken the immune response and increase susceptibility to infections and autoimmune diseases.

Metabolic Disorders Inflammatory molecules entering the bloodstream can interfere with metabolic processes, contributing to insulin resistance, weight gain, and an increased risk of type 2 diabetes. Alcohol's high caloric content and its effects on liver function exacerbate these risks.

Liver Damage The liver is responsible for detoxifying harmful substances that enter the bloodstream. When the gut barrier is compromised, the liver must work harder to process the influx of toxins and inflammatory molecules. Over time, this can lead to conditions such as fatty liver disease, alcoholic hepatitis, and cirrhosis.

Long-Term Health Consequences of Gut Permeability

Chronic alcohol consumption and the resulting gut permeability are linked to numerous long-term health problems. Beyond the immediate effects on brain function, immunity, and metabolism, leaky gut syndrome contributes to the development of several chronic diseases:

Cardiovascular Disease Inflammation triggered by gut leakage can damage blood vessels and increase the risk of atherosclerosis, hypertension, and heart attacks.

Neurodegenerative Disorders Persistent inflammation and the migration of toxins to the brain are associated with conditions such as Alzheimer's disease and Parkinson's disease.

Autoimmune Conditions The immune system's overreaction to harmful substances in the bloodstream may increase the risk of autoimmune disorders like rheumatoid arthritis, lupus, and celiac disease.

The connection between alcohol, gut permeability, and overall health underscores the importance of mindful consumption and proactive gut care. Alcohol's impact on the gut barrier can lead to a cascade of health issues, from chronic inflammation to neurological disorders. By reducing alcohol intake and adopting lifestyle habits that support gut health, individuals can improve their physical, mental, and emotional well-being. Protecting the gut is not just about avoiding disease; it is a foundational step toward achieving optimal health and vitality.

Disrupted Sleep Cycles

Case Study #25: The microbiome affects melatonin production, which regulates sleep. Alcohol-induced dysbiosis disrupts this process, leading to poor sleep quality.

The microbiome, a community of trillions of bacteria, fungi, and other microorganisms residing primarily in the gut, plays a critical role in regulating various aspects of human health. One of its lesser-known yet essential functions is its influence on melatonin production. Melatonin, often referred to as the "sleep hormone," is crucial for maintaining our sleep-wake cycle, also known as the circadian rhythm. When the microbiome is in a balanced state, it supports the production of melatonin and fosters healthy sleep patterns. However, when disrupted by factors such as alcohol consumption, this process can be severely impaired.

Melatonin is primarily produced by the pineal gland in the brain, but a significant portion of it is also synthesized in the gut, where the microbiome resides. The gut and brain communicate through the gut-brain axis, a bidirectional signaling pathway that involves hormones, neurotransmitters, and the nervous system. The health of the microbiome is therefore closely linked to sleep quality, making it a key area of focus for improving sleep and overall well-being.

The gut microbiome influences melatonin production through several mechanisms. One of the most important ways it does this is by aiding in the synthesis of serotonin, a neurotransmitter that serves as a precursor to melatonin. Serotonin is produced in the gut in response to the presence of specific beneficial bacteria. Without these bacteria, the production of serotonin and subsequently melatonin can be compromised, leading to disruptions in the sleep-wake cycle.

Another important mechanism involves the interaction between the gut microbiome and the immune system. A healthy microbiome produces metabolites such as short-chain fatty acids (SCFAs), which have anti-inflammatory properties and support the integrity of the gut lining. This helps prevent systemic inflammation that could otherwise interfere with the production of melatonin and disrupt sleep. Furthermore, certain gut bacteria can directly metabolize dietary nutrients into compounds that stimulate the synthesis of melatonin in the gut.

When the microbiome is balanced and diverse, it creates an environment conducive to stable melatonin production. This, in turn, helps regulate the circadian rhythm, ensuring restful and restorative sleep. Conversely, when the microbiome is thrown out of balance, known as dysbiosis, it can disrupt these processes and contribute to sleep disturbances.

Alcohol consumption is one of the leading causes of gut dysbiosis, a condition characterized by an imbalance in the gut microbiome. Alcohol can damage the intestinal lining, increase gut permeability (commonly known as "leaky gut"), and reduce the diversity of beneficial bacteria. This disruption has far-reaching consequences, including its impact on melatonin production and sleep quality.

When alcohol is consumed, it creates a hostile environment for beneficial gut bacteria while promoting the growth of harmful bacteria and fungi. This imbalance can *decrease the production of serotonin and melatonin, leading to disrupted sleep patterns.* Alcohol also increases systemic inflammation, which can further interfere with melatonin synthesis. Chronic alcohol consumption exacerbates these effects, creating a vicious cycle of poor gut health and poor sleep quality.

Moreover, alcohol affects the liver's ability to process and eliminate toxins efficiently. This can lead to the accumulation of harmful substances in the body, which further disrupts the gut-brain axis.

The resulting inflammation and oxidative stress can impair the brain's ability to regulate sleep, compounding the negative effects of alcohol-induced dysbiosis.

Poor sleep quality has a cascade of negative effects on physical and mental health. When sleep is disrupted due to alcohol-induced dysbiosis, it can lead to a range of issues, including fatigue, impaired cognitive function, mood disturbances, and weakened immune function. Over time, chronic sleep deprivation increases the risk of developing serious health conditions such as cardiovascular disease, diabetes, and obesity.

Sleep is a time for the body to repair and regenerate. During deep sleep, the brain clears out metabolic waste products, the immune system strengthens its defenses, and cells throughout the body undergo repair processes. When sleep is compromised, these critical functions are hindered, leading to long-term health consequences.

Alcohol and Obesity

Case Study #26: A study in *Obesity Reviews* linked alcohol consumption to changes in gut microbiota that promote weight gain and hinder fat metabolism.

When discussing factors that contribute to weight gain, alcohol is often overlooked. However, a growing body of research highlights its significant role in altering the gut microbiome in ways that encourage weight gain and disrupt fat metabolism. These findings shed light on why alcohol consumption might be more detrimental to maintaining a healthy weight than previously understood.

The gut microbiome is a complex ecosystem of trillions of bacteria, fungi, and other microorganisms living in our digestive tract. These microbes are essential for various bodily functions, including digestion, immune system support, and the production of vital compounds. One of their most critical roles is regulating metabolism, including how the body stores and burns fat.

When the gut microbiome is balanced, it helps maintain healthy energy levels and supports weight management. However, disruptions to this delicate balance, known as dysbiosis, can lead to an array of metabolic issues, including weight gain, inflammation, and impaired fat metabolism. Alcohol consumption has emerged as a significant disruptor of gut health, with far-reaching consequences for the body's ability to maintain a healthy weight.

Alcohol affects the gut microbiome in several ways. First, it reduces microbial diversity, meaning fewer types of beneficial bacteria thrive in the gut. Studies have shown that a diverse microbiome is essential for robust metabolic health, as different bacteria perform unique and complementary roles in digestion and fat regulation.

In addition to reducing diversity, alcohol promotes the growth of harmful bacteria such as *Proteobacteria*, which are linked to inflammation and metabolic disorders. This imbalance creates a hostile environment that impairs the gut's ability to process and metabolize fats efficiently. Over time, these changes can make it more challenging for the body to burn fat, leading to increased fat storage and, consequently, weight gain.

Moreover, alcohol damages the intestinal lining, leading to a condition often referred to as "leaky gut." This allows harmful substances, including bacterial toxins, to enter the bloodstream, triggering systemic inflammation. Chronic inflammation is closely associated with obesity and a reduced ability to burn fat.

One of the most concerning effects of alcohol on the gut microbiota is its role in hindering fat metabolism. The body's ability to break down and utilize fat efficiently is essential for weight management. Alcohol disrupts this process in several ways:

Redirection of Energy Pathways When alcohol is consumed, the body prioritizes metabolizing it over other energy sources, including fat. This means that for 24 to 48 hours after drinking alcohol, fat burning is effectively paused. During this time, the body stores fat instead of using it for energy.

Microbial Influence on Fat Storage Certain gut bacteria are associated with increased fat storage. When alcohol disrupts the balance of the gut microbiota, it encourages the proliferation of these fat-storing bacteria, further compounding weight gain.

Increased Lipogenesis Alcohol consumption stimulates a process known as de novo lipogenesis, where the liver converts excess carbohydrates and alcohol into fat. This newly created fat is stored in the body, often around the abdomen, contributing to visceral fat accumulation.

The Link Between Alcohol, Sugar Cravings, and Overeating

Another way alcohol contributes to weight gain is by altering gut bacteria in a manner that increases sugar cravings and appetite. *Certain bacteria in the gut communicate with the brain through the gut-brain axis, influencing hunger and food preferences.* Alcohol-induced dysbiosis can enhance the presence of bacteria that thrive on sugar and carbohydrates, leading to stronger cravings for these foods.

By disrupting the gut's delicate balance, alcohol not only promotes weight gain but also sets the stage for broader metabolic challenges, including inflammation and reduced fat metabolism.

Recognizing these effects allows individuals to make more informed choices about their alcohol consumption. For those seeking to manage their weight or improve their overall health, reducing or eliminating alcohol may be a pivotal step. Combined with other lifestyle changes that support gut health, it is possible to reverse the damage and create a foundation for long-term wellness.

The connection between alcohol and the gut microbiome is a reminder of how interconnected our bodies are. Small changes, such as cutting back on alcohol and incorporating gut-friendly foods, can lead to significant improvements in weight management and metabolic health. By prioritizing gut health, individuals can break free from the cycle of weight gain and enjoy a healthier, more balanced life.

Behavioral Changes Driven by Gut Microbes

Case Study #27: Microbiome alterations caused by alcohol have been shown to influence behavior, increasing risk-taking and impulsivity.

A growing body of research has begun to uncover the significant ways in which alcohol consumption impacts gut health. These discoveries shed light on the complex relationship between alcohol, gut bacteria, and overall metabolic health, offering important insights into why cutting back on alcohol could play a pivotal role in maintaining a healthy weight.

The gut microbiota refers to the trillions of microorganisms that reside in the gastrointestinal tract, including bacteria, viruses, fungi, and other microbes. These tiny organisms play a vital role in human health, aiding in digestion, nutrient absorption, immune system function, and even mental well-being. A balanced gut microbiota supports metabolic health by helping the body process nutrients efficiently and by regulating hormones that influence hunger, fat storage, and energy expenditure. However, when this delicate balance is disrupted, it can lead to a range of health issues, including obesity and metabolic disorders.

Alcohol consumption is known to have a profound impact on the composition and function of the gut microbiota. Studies have found that alcohol disrupts the balance of beneficial and harmful bacteria in the gut, a condition known as dysbiosis. Dysbiosis occurs when the population of beneficial microbes decreases while harmful bacteria multiply, leading to inflammation and other negative effects on gut health.

One of the ways alcohol promotes dysbiosis is by damaging the gut lining. Alcohol increases intestinal permeability, often referred to as "leaky gut." This condition allows harmful substances like toxins and bacteria to enter the bloodstream, triggering systemic inflammation. Chronic inflammation, in turn, is a known contributor to weight gain and difficulty in losing fat. Moreover, alcohol alters the types of bacteria present in the gut, favoring those associated with fat storage and increased calorie extraction from food. This means that even without consuming more calories, the body may store more fat when the gut microbiota is out of balance.

The study in *Obesity Reviews* highlights how alcohol's effects on gut bacteria directly contribute to weight gain. *Certain bacterial strains thrive in the presence of alcohol and produce byproducts that influence the body's ability to burn fat.* For instance, alcohol consumption has been linked to an increase in bacteria that produce lipopolysaccharides (LPS), molecules that trigger inflammation and impair metabolic processes. *High levels of LPS in the bloodstream are associated with insulin resistance,* which makes it harder for the body to use glucose for energy and encourages fat storage instead.

Additionally, wWhen alcohol is consumed, the liver prioritizes breaking down alcohol over other metabolic tasks, such as processing fats and carbohydrates. *This shift, which lasts for 24-48 hours after consuming alcohol, means that dietary fats stored rather than burned for energy.* Combined with the changes in gut bacteria, this creates a metabolic environment that favors weight gain and inhibits fat loss.

By disrupting the delicate balance of gut bacteria, alcohol creates an environment that promotes inflammation, impairs fat-burning processes, and encourages fat storage. These findings highlight the importance of considering gut health as a central factor in weight management strategies.

Delayed Liver Recovery

Case Study #28: Alcohol's prioritization in metabolism delays liver recovery, compounding the effects of fatty liver disease and other metabolic disorders.

When alcohol enters the body, it takes priority in the metabolic chain due to its toxicity. The human body lacks a storage mechanism for alcohol, unlike carbohydrates, fats, and proteins. This means alcohol must be metabolized immediately to prevent it from accumulating and causing damage to vital organs. While this prioritization is crucial for detoxifying the body, it comes at a cost: the delay of other essential metabolic processes. Over time, this disruption can exacerbate conditions like fatty liver disease and other metabolic disorders, highlighting the intricate and often harmful relationship between alcohol and metabolism.

The liver is the primary organ responsible for breaking down alcohol. When you drink, alcohol is absorbed through the stomach and intestines and then travels through the bloodstream to the liver. Here, specialized enzymes, primarily alcohol dehydrogenase (ADH) and aldehyde dehydrogenase (ALDH), begin the process of converting alcohol into acetaldehyde, a highly toxic compound, and then into acetate, a less harmful substance. Acetate is eventually broken down into water and carbon dioxide, which are expelled from the body.

This entire process requires significant energy and resources from the liver. While the liver is metabolizing alcohol, it temporarily halts the breakdown of fats and other nutrients. This delay forces the liver to store excess fat, contributing to the development of fatty liver disease over time. Repeated cycles of alcohol consumption and metabolism leave the liver in a constant state of catch-up, impairing its ability to recover and function optimally.

Fatty liver disease, also known as hepatic steatosis, occurs when excessive fat builds up in the liver. This condition is often the first stage of alcohol-related liver damage. Chronic alcohol consumption worsens fatty liver disease in several ways. First, as mentioned, the liver prioritizes alcohol metabolism over fat metabolism, leading to the accumulation of fat within its cells. Additionally, alcohol metabolism produces harmful byproducts like reactive oxygen species (ROS) and free radicals, which cause oxidative stress and damage liver cells. Over time, this cellular damage can progress into more severe conditions, such as alcoholic hepatitis or cirrhosis.

Another factor is the role of triglycerides. Alcohol increases the synthesis of triglycerides in the liver while simultaneously reducing the liver's ability to export these fats. The result is an overburdened liver, struggling to balance detoxification and fat management. Even for those who consume alcohol in moderation, consistent intake can contribute to the gradual development of fatty liver disease, especially when combined with a high-fat or high-sugar diet.

Beyond the liver, alcohol disrupts the metabolism of other macronutrients, which has a cascading effect on overall health. For instance, alcohol inhibits **gluconeogenesis**, the process by which the liver generates glucose from non-carbohydrate sources. This disruption can lead to unstable blood sugar levels, increasing the risk of hypoglycemia, particularly in individuals with diabetes or those who consume alcohol on an empty stomach.

Moreover, alcohol interferes with protein synthesis in the liver, which is essential for producing vital enzymes and proteins needed for repair and growth. Over time, these metabolic disruptions weaken the body's ability to heal itself, contributing to a range of metabolic disorders such as insulin resistance, obesity, and even cardiovascular disease. Alcohol consumption also alters the gut microbiome, which plays a critical role in regulating metabolism. An imbalanced gut microbiome can exacerbate inflammation and contribute to the development of metabolic syndrome.

Reducing alcohol intake offers far-reaching benefits for metabolic health. For starters, it allows the liver to prioritize the metabolism of fats, proteins, and carbohydrates, improving energy balance and reducing the risk of fatty liver disease. Over time, this can lead to better overall health, including stable blood sugar levels, improved cholesterol profiles, and reduced inflammation. Additionally, giving the liver time to recover enhances its ability to filter toxins, manage hormone levels, and regulate other vital processes.

Beyond the physical benefits, reducing alcohol consumption can also improve mental clarity, energy levels, and emotional well-being. Many individuals report feeling more focused and energized after cutting back on alcohol, as their bodies are no longer burdened by the constant cycle of detoxification. For those at risk of developing metabolic disorders, reducing alcohol can be a critical step in preventing long-term complications.

Alcohol's prioritization in metabolism is a survival mechanism that protects the body from immediate harm, because alcohol is a toxin and your body is working to expel the alcohol. However, this process comes at a significant cost to liver health and overall metabolic function. By prioritizing alcohol metabolism, the liver delays essential processes like fat breakdown and toxin removal, leading to the development of fatty liver disease and other metabolic disorders.

The good news is that the liver is a remarkable organ, capable of recovery when given the chance. By reducing alcohol intake, adopting a healthy lifestyle, and supporting the liver with nutrient-rich foods and hydration, individuals can break the cycle of damage and impaired recovery. Ultimately, understanding the relationship between alcohol and metabolism empowers individuals to make informed choices for their long-term health and well-being.

Altered Neural Pathways

Case Study #29: Studies in neuroscience journals highlight how alcohol-induced microbiome changes affect neural pathways associated with reward and addiction.

The relationship between the gut and the brain, often referred to as the gut-brain axis, is a complex communication network that significantly affects mental and physical health. Alcohol, a common social lubricant, disrupts this delicate system, *leading to changes that fuel addiction and cravings.*

The gut microbiome is a diverse community of trillions of microorganisms, including bacteria, fungi, and viruses, that reside in the gastrointestinal tract. This ecosystem plays an essential role in maintaining health, supporting digestion, modulating the immune system, and influencing brain function. A balanced microbiome promotes the production of neurotransmitters like serotonin, dopamine, and gamma-aminobutyric acid (GABA), which regulate mood, motivation, and stress response.

However, alcohol consumption can disrupt this balance. Excessive alcohol intake promotes the growth of harmful bacteria while reducing the population of beneficial microbes. This dysbiosis can result in systemic inflammation, compromised gut barrier integrity, and altered communication along the gut-brain axis. These changes set the stage for significant neural impacts, particularly in areas of the brain involved in reward and addiction.

Alcohol and the Reward Pathways

Alcohol directly influences the brain's reward system, a network of structures that include the nucleus accumbens, the prefrontal cortex, and the ventral tegmental area. These areas are rich in dopamine, the neurotransmitter associated with pleasure and reward. When alcohol is consumed, it triggers a release of dopamine, creating feelings of euphoria and reinforcing the behavior. Over time, repeated alcohol consumption hijacks this reward system, leading to dependence and addiction.

Recent neuroscience studies have revealed how alcohol-induced changes in the gut microbiome amplify this effect. Dysbiosis alters the production of short-chain fatty acids (SCFAs) and other metabolites that influence the brain's reward pathways. Harmful gut bacteria produce compounds that increase inflammation and stress hormone levels, both of which intensify cravings and reduce the brain's ability to regulate reward-seeking behaviors.

Inflammation: A Catalyst for Neural Changes

One of the most significant consequences of alcohol-induced gut dysbiosis is systemic inflammation. When the gut barrier is compromised, harmful substances like lipopolysaccharides (LPS) from bacterial cell walls enter the bloodstream. This triggers an immune response, leading to increased production of pro-inflammatory cytokines. These inflammatory molecules can cross the blood-brain barrier, impacting brain function.

Chronic inflammation in the brain, also known as neuroinflammation, affects the prefrontal cortex, which is responsible for decision-making, impulse control, and goal-directed behavior. Impaired functioning in this region can make it more difficult for individuals to resist cravings or make healthy choices. Additionally, inflammation disrupts the balance of neurotransmitters, further reinforcing addictive behaviors.

The Role of the Vagus Nerve in Gut-Brain Communication

The vagus nerve, a critical component of the gut-brain axis, acts as a communication superhighway between the gut and the brain. Signals from the gut microbiome travel along the vagus nerve, influencing mood, stress response, and reward processing. Alcohol-induced dysbiosis interferes with these signals, exacerbating the brain's vulnerability to addiction.

For example, beneficial gut bacteria produce metabolites that stimulate the vagus nerve to release anti-inflammatory signals and promote neurogenesis (the growth of new neurons). When these bacteria are diminished due to alcohol consumption, these protective effects are lost. Instead, harmful signals may dominate, contributing to mood disorders, anxiety, and heightened susceptibility to addictive behaviors.

Breaking the Cycle of Alcohol-Induced Changes

Understanding the interplay between alcohol, the gut microbiome, and neural pathways provides valuable insights into breaking the cycle of addiction. Restoring balance to the microbiome through dietary interventions, probiotics, and lifestyle changes can help mitigate the negative effects of alcohol on the brain. Key strategies include:

Adopting a Gut-Friendly Diet Incorporating fiber-rich foods, fermented products like yogurt and kimchi, and polyphenol-rich foods such as berries and green tea can promote the growth of beneficial gut bacteria.

Reducing Alcohol Intake Even moderate reductions in alcohol consumption can allow the gut to begin healing and reduce systemic inflammation.

Supplementing with Probiotics Certain probiotic strains, such as *Lactobacillus* and *Bifidobacterium*, have been shown to improve gut health and reduce inflammation.

Engaging in Regular Exercise Physical activity supports a healthy microbiome and improves mood-regulating brain chemicals.

Managing Stress Practices like mindfulness, meditation, and yoga can reduce stress and inflammation, supporting gut-brain communication.

Ongoing research in the fields of neuroscience and microbiome science continues to uncover new ways to address alcohol addiction through the gut-brain connection. Personalized medicine approaches that tailor interventions based on an individual's microbiome composition hold promise for more effective treatments. Additionally, advancements in prebiotics, postbiotics, and psychobiotics (bacteria that positively affect mental health) could revolutionize the way we approach addiction and recovery.

In conclusion, alcohol-induced changes in the gut microbiome have profound effects on neural pathways associated with reward and addiction. By disrupting the gut-brain axis, alcohol not only harms physical health but also reinforces cycles of craving and dependence. However, with a growing understanding of these mechanisms, there is hope for innovative strategies to restore balance and promote recovery.

Generational Impact

Case Study #30: Emerging research suggests that alcohol's impact on the microbiome can be passed to offspring, influencing their gut health and susceptibility to addiction.

Emerging scientific research has begun shedding light on a fascinating yet concerning phenomenon: the impact of alcohol consumption on the gut microbiome and how these effects can potentially be transmitted to future generations. The gut microbiome, a complex community of trillions of microorganisms residing in the digestive tract, plays a pivotal role in maintaining overall health, regulating metabolism, and even influencing brain function. When disrupted by external factors such as alcohol, the microbiome's balance can be thrown off, leading to far-reaching consequences not only for the individual but also for their offspring. This revelation raises important questions about the intergenerational effects of alcohol consumption and the steps that can be taken to mitigate these risks.

The gut microbiome is often referred to as the body's "second brain" due to its profound impact on physical and mental health.

Composed of diverse bacteria, viruses, fungi, and other microorganisms, this ecosystem contributes to digestion, immune function, and even mood regulation.

A balanced microbiome is essential for producing key neurotransmitters like serotonin and for preventing harmful pathogens from proliferating in the body. However, this delicate balance can be easily disturbed by diet, stress, medications, and, notably, alcohol consumption.

Alcohol is a known disruptor of the microbiome. Studies have shown that even moderate drinking can reduce microbial diversity in the gut, favoring the growth of harmful bacteria and reducing populations of beneficial ones. This imbalance, known as dysbiosis, can lead to inflammation, impaired digestion, and a weakened immune system. Over time, chronic alcohol use may cause more severe gut issues, such as leaky gut syndrome, where the intestinal lining becomes more permeable, allowing toxins and harmful microbes to enter the bloodstream. These changes don't only affect the individual but can also influence the health of their offspring in unexpected ways.

Alcohol and Epigenetic Changes in the Microbiome

The concept of epigenetics provides a key framework for understanding how alcohol's effects on the microbiome can be inherited. Epigenetics refers to changes in gene expression that do not involve alterations to the DNA sequence itself but are influenced by environmental factors. When alcohol disrupts the microbiome, it can trigger epigenetic modifications that alter how genes involved in gut health and metabolism are expressed.

These changes can then be passed down to offspring, potentially predisposing them to a range of health issues.

For example, research has demonstrated that alcohol-induced changes in gut bacteria can affect the development of the offspring's microbiome even before birth. The maternal microbiome, which heavily influences the colonization of the infant's gut during pregnancy and delivery, serves as a crucial link in this process. If a mother's microbiome has been compromised by alcohol consumption, her child may inherit a less diverse and less robust microbiome, increasing their susceptibility to digestive issues, immune dysfunction, and even mental health challenges later in life.

The Link Between Gut Health and Addiction Susceptibility

One of the most intriguing and troubling findings in recent research is the potential connection between alcohol's impact on the microbiome and an offspring's vulnerability to addiction. The gut-brain axis—a bidirectional communication network between the gut and the brain—plays a significant role in shaping behavior and emotional responses. Disruptions in the gut microbiome can influence the production of neurotransmitters and hormones that regulate mood, stress, and reward pathways in the brain.

When a child inherits a dysregulated microbiome due to parental alcohol consumption, their gut-brain axis may also be impaired. This disruption could make them more prone to anxiety, depression, or impulsive behaviors, all of which are risk factors for addiction. Additionally, certain harmful bacteria that thrive in alcohol-altered microbiomes may produce metabolites that mimic addictive substances, potentially priming the brain's reward system for addictive behaviors.

Animal studies have provided some of the strongest evidence for this connection. For instance, experiments with rodents have shown that offspring of alcohol-exposed parents exhibit altered microbiome profiles and are more likely to engage in addictive behaviors compared to those of non-exposed parents. While more research is needed to fully understand these mechanisms in humans, the implications are clear: parental alcohol consumption could have long-term effects on a child's risk of addiction.

Maternal and Paternal Contributions

The role of maternal microbiome health in shaping an infant's gut has been well-documented, but recent studies suggest that fathers may also contribute to this intergenerational transfer. Alcohol consumption in men can lead to changes in sperm that affect the genetic and epigenetic material passed to offspring.

These changes, combined with the father's influence on the household microbiome environment, may play a role in shaping the child's gut health and overall well-being.

In maternal cases, the transmission of a compromised microbiome begins during pregnancy and continues through childbirth and breastfeeding. The microbiota present in the birth canal and breast milk serve as key sources of microbial colonization for the infant. If alcohol has disrupted these microbial populations, the infant may receive a suboptimal foundation for their gut health. For fathers, while the mechanism is less direct, their contribution to the household's microbial environment—through shared living spaces and dietary habits—can influence the composition of their children's microbiome over time.

Strategies for Breaking the Cycle

Understanding the intergenerational effects of alcohol on the microbiome underscores the importance of preventive measures and proactive interventions. For individuals planning to have children, reducing or eliminating alcohol consumption can significantly improve the health of their microbiome, providing a better foundation for future generations. Here are several strategies to consider:

Adopting a Gut-Friendly Diet Consuming a diet rich in prebiotic and probiotic foods can help restore and maintain microbial balance. Foods like yogurt, kefir, fermented vegetables, and fiber-rich fruits and vegetables support the growth of beneficial bacteria.

Engaging in Alcohol-Free Periods Participating in alcohol-free challenges such as Dry January or Sober October allows the gut to heal and recover from the disruptive effects of alcohol. These periods can also help individuals develop healthier habits around alcohol consumption.

Using Probiotic Supplements High-quality probiotic supplements can introduce beneficial bacteria to the gut and help counteract dysbiosis. Consulting with a healthcare provider can ensure the right strains and dosages are selected.

Fostering a Healthy Household Microbiome Encouraging family members to adopt gut-healthy practices can create a supportive environment for microbial diversity. Shared activities like eating fermented foods, gardening, or spending time in nature can boost microbial exposure for everyone.

Educating About Epigenetics Raising awareness about the epigenetic implications of alcohol consumption can motivate individuals to make informed decisions that benefit not only themselves but also their potential children.

As research into the relationship between alcohol, the microbiome, and intergenerational health continues to evolve, it becomes increasingly clear that the choices individuals make today can have profound effects on future generations. The gut microbiome is a critical component of health, and its disruption through alcohol consumption is a preventable risk factor with far-reaching consequences.

By prioritizing gut health and understanding the epigenetic ripple effects of lifestyle choices, individuals can take meaningful steps to protect their own well-being and that of their children. The emerging science serves as both a warning and an opportunity: while alcohol's impact on the microbiome may seem daunting, it also provides a powerful motivation to adopt healthier habits that promote resilience and vitality for generations to come.

Summary

The gut-brain axis refers to the complex communication network linking the gastrointestinal tract (gut) and the central nervous system (brain). This bidirectional system allows the gut and brain to share information, coordinating physical and mental health. The connection operates through neural pathways, hormonal signals, and immune responses, making the gut a second brain of sorts. Central to this system is the vagus nerve, which transmits messages between the brain and the gut, allowing emotional states, hunger, and digestion to influence one another. Understanding the gut-brain axis is vital to addressing issues like addiction, as this relationship profoundly affects mood, behavior, and cravings.

Gut bacteria play a critical role in the gut-brain axis. The human gut houses trillions of microbes, collectively known as the gut microbiome. These microbes produce neurotransmitters like serotonin, dopamine, and gamma-aminobutyric acid (GABA), which influence mood and behavior. For example, about 90% of the body's serotonin—a key player in regulating mood—is produced in the gut. Disruptions in the microbiome can lead to imbalances in these chemicals, potentially driving behaviors associated with addiction.

Cravings, particularly for sugar and alcohol, can also be linked to the microbiome. Certain gut bacteria thrive on these substances and may manipulate neural pathways to signal cravings. These bacteria essentially "hijack" the gut-brain axis to ensure their survival, creating a feedback loop that reinforces unhealthy habits.

Gut dysbiosis—an imbalance between beneficial and harmful gut bacteria—is a common factor in addiction. When harmful bacteria outnumber the good ones, it disrupts the production of neurotransmitters and other chemical signals. This imbalance can exacerbate anxiety, depression, and other mental health issues, increasing vulnerability to addictive behaviors.

Moreover, gut dysbiosis can impair the body's ability to regulate blood sugar, leading to erratic energy levels and heightened cravings for quick sources of energy, such as sugar and alcohol. Addressing gut health is therefore crucial for breaking the cycle of addiction and restoring emotional and physical balance.

Sugar and alcohol cravings share a surprising commonality: both are influenced by the same reward pathways in the brain. Consuming these substances triggers the release of dopamine, the "feel-good" neurotransmitter, reinforcing their consumption. Interestingly, the gut microbiome also plays a role in these cravings. Certain bacteria that thrive on sugar can also metabolize alcohol, making individuals prone to simultaneous sugar and alcohol cravings. This connection explains why individuals with a history of excessive sugar consumption may find it harder to abstain from alcohol and vice versa.

Some gut bacteria—commonly referred to as "bad bugs"—depend on sugar and alcohol for their growth and survival. These microbes release metabolites that affect the gut-brain axis, signaling the brain to crave more of these substances.

For instance, Candida yeast, a type of fungus often associated with gut dysbiosis, thrives on sugar and alcohol. Over time, feeding these microbes creates a dependence that can fuel addiction and make it challenging to adopt healthier habits.

Feeding harmful microbes perpetuates a vicious cycle. When sugar or alcohol is consumed, these substances not only nourish the bad bugs but also suppress the growth of beneficial bacteria. This imbalance further disrupts the gut microbiome, intensifying cravings and reducing the body's resilience to stress and emotional triggers. Breaking this cycle requires targeted dietary and lifestyle changes to starve the bad bugs while promoting the growth of beneficial bacteria.

What Happens in Your Body After Consuming Alcohol

When you consume alcohol, your body prioritizes metabolizing it over other nutrients. Unlike carbohydrates, fats, and proteins, alcohol cannot be stored in the body, so it must be processed immediately. This process primarily occurs in the liver, where enzymes break down alcohol into acetaldehyde, a toxic compound, and then into acetate, which can be used as energy.

Why Your Body Prioritizes Metabolizing Alcohol Over Burning Fat

Alcohol is treated as a toxin by the body, making its elimination a top priority. While the liver metabolizes alcohol, other metabolic processes, such as fat oxidation, are temporarily put on hold. This prioritization disrupts the body's natural fat-burning processes, making it harder to lose weight.

After consuming alcohol, the body experiences a 24-48-hour hiatus from fat-burning. During this period, the liver focuses on processing alcohol, and the oxidation of fats and carbohydrates is significantly reduced. This interruption not only slows weight loss but also contributes to fat storage, particularly in the abdominal area. For individuals working on improving their metabolism or losing weight, understanding this pause in fat-burning can be a powerful motivator to limit alcohol consumption.

Foods to Feed "Good" Bacteria and Starve "Bad" Ones

Supporting the gut microbiome requires a diet rich in foods that nourish beneficial bacteria while discouraging the growth of harmful ones. Fiber-rich foods, such as fruits, vegetables, legumes, and whole grains, are excellent choices for feeding good bacteria. Certain "prebiotic" foods, like garlic, onions, and bananas, serve as fuel for these microbes, promoting a healthy balance in the gut.

Conversely, reducing sugar, processed foods, and alcohol is crucial for starving harmful bacteria. These substances feed bad bugs and exacerbate gut dysbiosis, making it harder to maintain a healthy microbiome.

Probiotics, Prebiotics, and Fermented Foods for Gut Health

Incorporating probiotics, prebiotics, and fermented foods into your diet can further support gut health. Probiotics are live bacteria found in foods like yogurt, kefir, and kimchi, which help replenish beneficial microbes. Prebiotics, found in foods like asparagus and leeks, provide nourishment for these bacteria. Fermented foods, such as sauerkraut and miso, offer a dual benefit of probiotics and digestive enzymes, aiding gut repair and overall health.

Evidence-Based Methods to Reduce Cravings

Stabilizing blood sugar levels is a key strategy for reducing cravings. Eating balanced meals that combine complex carbohydrates, lean proteins, and healthy fats can prevent spikes and crashes in blood sugar, reducing the urge for quick fixes like sugar or alcohol. Whole foods like sweet potatoes, quinoa, and avocados provide sustained energy and support gut health.

Fiber, protein, and healthy fats play a significant role in managing cravings. Fiber slows digestion, prolonging feelings of fullness and stabilizing blood sugar. Protein provides a steady source of energy, while healthy fats, like those found in nuts and olive oil, promote satiety. Incorporating these nutrients into meals and snacks can help break the cycle of cravings.

Mindful eating involves being fully present during meals, paying attention to hunger and fullness cues, and savoring each bite. This practice can reduce emotional eating, which often drives sugar and alcohol cravings. Addressing emotional triggers through therapy, journaling, or meditation can also help individuals develop healthier coping mechanisms.

How Gut Health Influences Brain Function and Mental Clarity

A healthy gut is essential for optimal brain function and mental clarity. The gut produces key neurotransmitters that affect focus, memory, and mood. Dysbiosis can lead to inflammation and "brain fog," impairing cognitive abilities and emotional stability. Improving gut health can enhance mental clarity and support overall well-being.

Healing the gut involves dietary changes, stress management, and targeted supplementation. Eating a nutrient-dense diet, incorporating probiotics, and reducing stress through practices like yoga or deep breathing can repair the gut lining and restore balance to the microbiome. These steps can significantly improve focus and mood stability.

How Fasting Kills Off Bad Bacteria That Cause Dysbiosis

Fasting creates an environment in the gut that is less hospitable to harmful bacteria. By depriving these microbes of their preferred food sources, such as sugar and refined carbohydrates, fasting can reduce their population and restore balance to the microbiome. Autophagy, a process triggered by fasting, helps the body remove damaged cells and harmful bacteria, promoting overall gut health.

There are several types of fasting, each with its unique benefits. Intermittent fasting involves cycling between periods of eating and fasting, while prolonged fasting extends for 24 hours or more. Time-restricted eating limits food consumption to a specific window each day, such as 8 hours.

These methods can be tailored to individual needs and health goals. However, fasting is not suitable for everyone. Pregnant or breastfeeding women, individuals with a history of eating disorders, and those with certain medical conditions, such as diabetes or hypoglycemia, should consult a healthcare professional before attempting fasting. It is essential to ensure that fasting is safe and appropriate for individual circumstances.

To start fasting, gradually increase the fasting window over time to allow your body to adjust. Staying hydrated and consuming nutrient-dense meals during eating periods can support energy levels and prevent nutrient deficiencies. Listening to your body and breaking the fast with light, easily digestible foods is also important.

Building a Gut-Healthy Lifestyle for Sustainable Well-Being

Creating a lifestyle that supports gut health involves consistent dietary and lifestyle choices. Eating whole, unprocessed foods, managing stress, getting regular exercise, and prioritizing sleep are foundational habits for maintaining a balanced microbiome. These practices not only support gut health but also promote long-term physical and mental well-being, reducing the risk of addiction and other health issues.

Empower Your Microbiome, Empower Your Life

As we close this journey into the remarkable world of the microbiome and its influence on your cravings, health, and well-being, it's clear that healing your gut is about more than just diet—it's about reclaiming your power. The microbiome is a dynamic, living community that shapes the way you think, feel, and even crave. By supporting it, you can break free from the cycle of alcohol and sugar cravings that undermine your health.

Start by nourishing your microbiome with foods that foster good bacteria: fiber-rich vegetables, fermented foods like kimchi and kefir, and prebiotic staples such as garlic, onions, and bananas. These choices feed the good bacteria and crowd out the harmful ones that may be manipulating your gut-brain axis.

For those who can, intermittent fasting can be a transformative tool. It gives your digestive system a reset, promotes autophagy (your body's cellular clean-up process), and supports the balance of microbes in your gut. Even short fasting windows can make a difference when practiced mindfully.

Finally, avoid alcohol—not just as a short-term detox but as a gift to your gut. Alcohol disrupts the delicate microbial balance, feeding harmful bacteria and perpetuating the cravings that sabotage your goals. The more you avoid it, the stronger and healthier your microbiome becomes, enabling you to regain control over your cravings and your choices.

Healing your microbiome is not an overnight fix, but every step you take moves you closer to a life free from the grip of alcohol and sugar cravings. Your gut has an incredible capacity to heal when given the right tools. By nurturing it with the right foods, thoughtful fasting, and a commitment to avoiding substances that harm it, you're building a foundation for long-term health, clarity, and freedom.

This journey is yours to own. Embrace it, and let your microbiome become your greatest ally in the pursuit of a healthier, more vibrant life.